WORKING IN RESIDENTIAL HOMES FOR ELDERLY PEOPLE

In recent years there have been many changes in residential provisions for elderly people. The number of privately run homes has increased significantly, and there is a greater variety in size and type of home, offering consumers a wider choice. Paul Brearley's earlier book, *Residential Work with the Elderly* (1977), has been widely used by residential workers, and in this new book he provides another wide-ranging and helpful introduction to good practice and management.

Drawing on his extensive practical experience of social work and residential care, the author outlines the purposes and objectives of homes and what it is like to live and work in them. He looks at the factors that make for a good quality of life, considering how these can be promoted and how staff can work with people, both individually and in groups, to help them get the best out of life. He reviews current thinking about what happens to people as they grow older, and, at a practical level, he looks carefully at the day-to-day management of homes, suggesting how they should be organized in order to get the best out of staff, buildings, and resources.

Unique in its coverage of the process of ageing, good practice, and good management, *Working in Residential Homes for Elderly People* takes into account the differing needs of both residents and staff. With its emphasis on the various aspects of the flexible, individual support necessary in providing 'a good home', it will be invaluable to social work and social care students, residential workers, and their managers.

The author
Paul Brearley, writing in a personal capacity, is Assistant Chief Inspector, Social Services Inspectorate of the Department of Health.

WORKING IN RESIDENTIAL HOMES FOR ELDERLY PEOPLE

C. PAUL BREARLEY

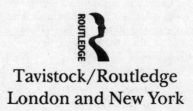

Tavistock/Routledge
London and New York

First published 1990
by Routledge
11 New Fetter Lane, London EC4P 4EE

Simultaneously published in the USA and Canada by Routledge
a division of Routledge, Chapman and Hall, Inc.
29 West 35th Street, New York, NY 10001

© 1990 C. Paul Brearley

Typeset by LaserScript Limited, Mitcham, Surrey
Printed and bound in Great Britain by
Biddles Ltd, Guildford and King's Lynn

British Library Cataloguing in Publication Data

Brearley, C. Paul (Christopher Paul), *1946–*
Working in residential homes for elderly people.
1. Old persons. Residential care
I. Title
362.6'1

Library of Congress Cataloging in Publication Data

Brearley, C. Paul.
Working in residential homes for elderly people /
C. Paul Brearley.
p.   cm.
Includes bibliographical references.
1. Old age homes–United States–Management. 2. Aged–
Institutional care–United States. 3. Social work with the aged–
United States. I. Title.
HV1454.2.U6B74   1990   89–77321
362.6'1'068–dc20   CIP

ISBN 0-415-03768-9
0-415-03769-7 (pbk)

CONTENTS

AUTHOR'S NOTE

Please note that the contents of this book represent the views of the author alone and in no way commit the Department of Health.

Chapter One

BEGINNING AT THE BEGINNING

There is a story about a manufacturing company which made chocolate-flavoured dessert. It decided to bow to the pressures of changing times and customer preferences. The description 'chocolate-flavoured' means, of course, that there was no chocolate: the flavour was created by additives. The company was under pressure to remove the additives. After extensive research and testing the experts were still unable to produce a chocolate flavour from less toxic additives. Eventually an innocent observer asked whether they had considered cocoa. Not only did this provide a chocolate-flavoured answer – it proved to be cheaper!

The moral of the story is perhaps that we need to go back to basics to find the best way to achieve our objectives. This is certainly so for residential Homes.

This consideration of residential provisions for elderly people needs to begin by asking what we want to achieve and for whom we want to achieve it. Then we can go on to look at the best ways of setting out to produce the results people need and want.

PEOPLE AND PLACES

That is, of course, easier said than done. People are very different and need different things at different times. Consider, for instance, the following snapshot descriptions:

Mr Andrews is 77 years old and lives in a Local Authority residential Home. He worked as a miner until retirement. Two of his three sons, who all live within a few miles of the Home, are also in the coal industry. His wife died three years ago. Physically he is still quite fit and walks considerable distances to do shopping for other residents. He starts the day cheerful and able to hold a reasonable conversation. As the day progresses his ideas become increasingly muddled. By evening he can sometimes be very confused and has been very aggressive and violent in his frustration. At night he is often restless and demanding.

Miss Baker is 94 and lives in a well-established privately-run Home. She has lived there for 15 years. She was a school teacher and latterly headmistress of a local school. She has no living relatives and since the death of a niece two years ago has had no visitors. Around the same time her capital ran low and she has been claiming state benefits since then. This is not sufficient to meet the full charge of the Home and some of her personal allowance has to be paid. She is very anxious and unhappy about this and sometimes appears forgetful and confused.

Mr Carter is 65 and lives in a Local Authority Home. He spent 20 years in the oil industry, much of that time in South America. He returned to the UK about ten years ago when his marriage ended in divorce. He had substantial funds which were rapidly depleted by his addiction to alcohol. At 64 he suffered a stroke which left him able to walk only with difficulty. As he has no one to support him he came into the Home where he feels misplaced and alone. He is eager to find somewhere else to live but staff feel he could not manage alone and find his continuing use of alcohol a problem to cope with in the Home.

Mrs Davies is 84 years old. A widow, she came into the Home a year ago following the amputation of her left leg below the knee. She uses a wheelchair, can dress herself (given time) but needs help in transferring from the chair to bed or toilet. One of her two daughters lives nearby: she visits regularly and Mrs Davies goes to her house for the day most Sundays. She shares a room with a lady who has been a distant acquaintance in the village for many years but who is now very confused. Mrs Davies gives her a lot of help but sometimes feels angry and frustrated at her behaviour.

These four people illustrate immediately some of the difficulties of trying to make a single prescription for the needs of 'old people' as if they were all the same or even similar. The age span alone shows that we must think in terms of varied solutions. At the end of the 1980s a woman of 94 may look back on the First World War as one of the most significant times of her life. A man in his mid-sixties will have been caught up in the later part of the Second World War. For others, the 1920s or 1930s will have been of greater significance. It is as well to remember that some people who have been grouped together as 'old' in residential care are old enough to be the parents of others in the same Home.

The places in which they find themselves living also have their own range and variety. For example:

Green Park is a new development on the outskirts of a large conurbation. It is an open-plan estate with a variety of small housing units, including flats and a few bungalows. All are for retired people. On the ten-acre site there is a private residential Home providing for 35 people. A call system links the houses to a central office in the residential Home. Help is available in emergencies.

The Manor is a large house, built in 1910 and bought and adapted by the Local Authority in 1957. There are two bedrooms which accommodate three people each: the rest are double rooms. The Council has considered selling the Home to a private company, resulting in considerable political hostility and a lot of anxiety for the present residents.

52, The Avenue is a large 1950s-built house on a residential estate. A year ago the owners converted a double garage and intended to provide for six elderly residents. They had planning permission but had not discussed their plans with the Social Services Department who are resisting granting registration. Three older people currently live there and receive substantial state benefits to meet their costs.

Harry Smith House was built by the Local Authority in 1963 and named after the then Leader of the Council. There are three large, central lounges next to each other. Bedrooms are in a series of wings radiating from the centre. The exterior is badly in need of decoration. The interior is uniformly painted, several rooms needing urgent redecoration. There are some carpets on the floor – some in bedrooms, some on corridors – but with no apparent logic to where they are; some residents have bought their own. There are 46 residents; most are women. Their average age is 83; the youngest is 73. Almost half appear to have some degree of confusion or mental disorder but few have been assessed by a psychiatrist. Few are able to walk outside the Home. Every week one or two new residents appear for a 'short stay': few of the established residents pay them any more than irritable attention.

Church House is a group of 30 flatlets. Most have one bedroom, a kitchenette, lounge and bathroom. A few are slightly larger. There is a lounge available to all the tenants with a kitchen, launderette and drying room. A warden lives in one of the flats and visits each tenant every morning and evening. She provides little practical help but will assist with arrangements at times of particular difficulty (calling the doctor, family or Social Services, occasionally helping with shopping during illness). The flats are owned by a small housing association.

Fairfields was built in the mid-1980s, financed jointly by a Social Services Department and District Health Authority. It provides ten single bedsitting rooms. Five of these are used for short stays for a variety of purposes. The other five are used to provide assessment stays, supported by the local Primary Health Care Team. There is a day-care facility which can accommodate up to 15 at a time. The kitchen provides meals-on-wheels. Social workers and home care workers are also based at the unit which has a manager with overall responsibility for all these services. The unit provides for the elderly people of a defined locality in which it is centrally based.

These examples begin to show the range of types of accommodation that have developed to provide for groups of elderly people together. The Registered Homes Act (1984) defined a residential Home. Basically it was defined for the purposes of registration with a regulating and controlling Local Authority as a place where four or more people receive both board and personal care. What makes a place 'a home' is not so easily defined. This will be considered in more detail later.

The important point, for the present, is that the term 'residential Home' covers a multitude of places and provisions for many very different people who are looking for very different things.

Since this is the case it is necessary to start from a very broad, preliminary base to 'begin with the basics'. The starting-point has to be with the nature and meaning of the experience of ageing and with the attitudes we all hold to ageing which underlie our expectations of the provisions we need to make.

AGEING AND ATTITUDES

The trouble with stereotypes is that, by definition, people believe them: a stereotype is a fixed and unchanging belief. There are a number of common stereotypes about ageing and old age. What we know about ageing is still very closely bound up with what we believe about it. This is complicated by the variety of words we use: age, ageing, aged, old, older, elderly, elders, etc.

Stereotypes of old age, sometimes called 'myths', are often contradictory. One common stereotype sees old age as a time of peace, tranquillity and relaxation after a lifetime of work. Old people are seen as wise, calm and reliable. On the other hand, there is a common belief that old people are likely to be rigid in their views, unwilling to change, 'senile', with irreversible mental and physical disease.

Both of these images represent extremes, some parts of which may be true for some people. There will, however, be considerable differences between the individual's experience of the ageing process and the standardized assumptions made by society. Difficulties arise because of the effects that societies have on individual behaviour and opportunity, both in the ways that an elderly person expects to behave and in the pressures created by those around her.

The word 'ageism' has been increasingly used since it was first coined in the mid-1970s to describe the process of stereotyping of older people and the discrimination that results. Explanations which have been offered for ageism usually suggest that it arises from a mixture of motivations. On the one hand, there are said to be aspects of ageing – such as the loss of strength and deterioration in energies and other abilities – which we prefer not to think about, so elderly people tend to be avoided because they are reminders of these things. On the other hand, we expect to grow old and to need the help and support of others when we do so. There is a mixture, therefore, of care and concern and fear and rejection in attitudes to age, ageing and 'the elderly'.

It is easy to produce a collection of facts to prove an apparently (but probably stereotypically) negative side of ageing. For instance:

- almost 70 per cent of disabled adults are aged 60 or over and almost half of all people with disabilites are over 70 (Martin *et al.* 1988);
- almost a third of people over 65 live alone;
- 44 per cent of people over 85 live alone;
- four out of five elderly people living alone are women: more than one third are women over 75;
- a quarter of all elderly people are widowed and living alone: a third of these will have been alone for at least ten years (Hunt 1978).

For women in particular old age is represented as an especially negative time:

> for most women, ageing means a humiliating process of gradual sexual disqualification. Since women are considered maximally eligible in early youth, after which their sexual value drops steadily, even young women feel themselves in a desperate race against the calendar.
>
> (Sontag 1972)

There is, however, another side to the coin:

- 76 per cent of people between 60 and 69 and almost 60 per cent of those between 70 and 79 do not report any disability (Martin *et al.* 1988);
- seven out of ten elderly people do live in shared households;
- more than half of those aged 85 and over live with at least one other person;
- 19 out of 20 have a close relative living and a third can expect

to be visited by relatives several times a week: a further quarter at least once a week;

- over 70 per cent are visited by friends and well over half visit friends in return (Hunt 1978).

A balanced view of age must consider both sides of the coin. There are difficulties for some elderly people at any point in time but most live a comfortable, satisfying life with the support of relatives and friends for whom they provide support and services in return. Only around 5 per cent of elderly people are in communal or institutional care and perhaps 13 per cent are largely housebound. Over 80 per cent, therefore, lead a more or less active life in the community.

Unfortunately, some of the negative attitudes of ageism are shared by professionals who work with elderly people. It is not surprising that this should be so. There is evidence that social workers, for example, feel that elderly people have 'had their chance' and have little further contribution to make to society. This is associated with a belief that elderly people as a group are less valuable than children. The tendency is, therefore, to focus on work with children who are seen to be both at greater risk and to offer greater potential for change.

Several factors are likely to influence the views of those who work with elderly people:

- assumptions that there is less hope of change with this group ('failure models');
- the low status of elderly people within society is reflected in the status of those who work with them and who themselves tend to be undervalued;
- the lack of specialist training in work with this group;
- the reality of high demand for limited resources which means that often not enough can be done to help;
- elderly people are nearer to death and are a reminder of mortality.

As Alison Norman has expressed it:

there is an ambivalence at the root of our being. Personal affection, a sense of duty, a desire not to hurt or reject and a deeply-conditioned belief in the value of individual life impel

7

us to honour, protect and defend... But there are other feelings... contempt of the young and strong for the old and weak; fear of the mortality which old age represents; guilt which is translated into action; and resentment over the need to use scarce resources and precious time on people who 'have had their life'.

(Norman 1987: 3)

But ageism and its potential influence on the way help is provided are not inevitable. What is needed is a balanced view of the realistic potential for helping elderly people to lead an active and satisfying life. Above all, we need a recognition of the individuality of each person and his or her unique needs.

ON 'LEARNING TO SPIT': THE INDIVIDUAL PERSPECTIVE

There are several ways to begin to 'understand' what ageing is all about. We can draw from research, or from the theoretical writings of the growing numbers of gerontologists or from the insights from literature. We can also look to the accounts of elderly people themselves: those who are closest to the experience.

Of course, people can only write of their experience of age if they see themselves as growing old. In a lively book about the nature and experience of ageing, Mary Stott says:

We are not old. As Bernard Baruch is reported to have said, 'old is always fifteen years older than I am'. We are young to ourselves most of our lives, young to our elders as long as we have any. A friend of eighty-one, knowing from her son of the way I over-filled my sixties with activities said fondly, 'What it is to be young'. Perhaps by seventy one is finding, disconcertingly, that people express no surprise when one says 'Of course I'm getting old'. There may come a day, in our late eighties perhaps, when we shall actually brag about our age. I don't know about that yet. 'Old' is fifteen years older than I am.

(Stott 1981: 176)

This vividly illustrates a key difference between *growing older*, a process of change through time which we can all understand and recognize, and *being older*, a much more difficult (and personal)

8

thing to define. The often-quoted poem attributed to Phyllis McCormack, angered at seeing the treatment of an elderly resident in a residential home, illustrates the difference between the ageing body and the feelings and awareness of the person within the body:

> What do you see nurses what do you see
> What are you thinking when you look at me?
> A crabbed old woman, not very wise
> Uncertain of habit, with faraway eyes. . .
> But inside this old carcass a young girl still dwells
> And now and again my battered heart swells,
> I remember the joys, I remember the pain,
> And I'm loving and living life over again.
> (McCormack, date unknown)

A more light-hearted view can be found in Jenny Joseph's poem 'Warning':

> When I am an old woman I shall wear purple
> With a red hat which doesn't go and doesn't suit me
> And I shall spend my pension on brandy and summer
>   gloves . . .
> I shall go out in my slippers in the rain
> And pick the flowers in other people's gardens
> And learn to spit.
> (Joseph 1974)

Not surprisingly, most personal accounts reflect a diversity of experience. When herself aged 80, Kathleen Gibberd wrote:

> Seen from the inside old age is not merely a downhill process. In reality it is an up-and-down affair, rather like a mountain descent where one finds oneself sometimes on a sunny plateau and then on a new and exhilarating height.
> (Gibberd 1977: 2)

This should be familiar to all who work with elderly people: their moods, expectations and wishes change from day to day. But is this only so for elderly people? Are we not all changeable? For some elderly people fluctuations in health and energy levels do lead to more noticeable changes than amongst many younger people.

There have been a number of recent books which have provided insights through records of interviews with elderly people. Jeremy Seabrook, for instance, provides extracts from his conversations with 21 elderly people about what they felt were the needs of 'the old'. The answers are diverting and illuminating. He concludes that what emerged more than anything was a 'wistfulness in relation to children'(Seabrook 1980: 118):

> Mr Hawtry. . . I don't like going home. It isn't a home, not for me. I live with my son and his wife and their kiddies. . . I wish I'd never given up mine. . . Ken always said to me and mother that which ever was left would always have a home with him. Lodger more like. . .
>
> (ibid.: 28)

> Mr Bunce. . . I grew up to expect the young to want to look after the old. They don't think they have any responsibility to me. I think they care for me, in their way. Its just that they don't realize that you need a bit of cherishing when you get old.
>
> (ibid.: 83)

Seabrook identifies, in particular, the ways in which the elderly people described their non-material needs (excluding health needs) as:

- the importance of company, being wanted and needed;
- the need for a sense of purpose or useful activity;
- a religious belief, 'peace of mind' or feeling an 'inner satisfaction';
- to have no needs beyond material needs.

These are reflected in the comments of other writers. Margery Fry was herself aged 80 when she wrote,

> Those who have learned to live (on however humble a scale) amongst the things of the mind can follow them more peacefully when instinct and ambition and competition are less disturbing and when leisure is compulsory.
>
> (Fry 1954: 10)

In a collection of descriptions of the lives of elderly women Ford and Sinclair (1987) put stronger emphasis on 'the structural

10

poverty and dependence that women experience and . . . the power of stereotypes that create a pervasive ageism in society' (p.7). They do conclude, however, that the values which guide the thinking of older people undergo a fundamental change. The goals of the women they interviewed were found to be the wish to strike a balance between the need for security and the need for independence and self-respect:

> Life's pleasures change as circumstances change. Mrs Patel still loves the noise and laughter her grandchildren bring but Mrs Harman now prefers the company of people her own age. . . Miss Moss enjoys the pleasures of not having to get up in the morning. Mrs Walls craves activities. . . Miss Stewart 'loves her telly'. When talking about what it was they were seeking from old age the women used phrases such as 'having some pleasure', 'peace', 'meeting people', 'enjoyment', 'pleasing myself', 'not having to fight'.

This sums up, perhaps, what we need to be aware of. A good old age is likely to include:

- material comfort (in the eye of the beholder!);
- good health;
- companionship, and contact with family and friends;
- a feeling of being useful, or of purposefulness;
- a feeling of satisfaction, pleasure or contentment.

What leads to satisfaction will be considered again in the next chapter. It should be clear from these extracts that it will be different for different people.

BACK TO BASICS: THE 'WHY' AND THE 'HOW'

This, then, is the basic: there can be no universal solutions. People need individual opportunities and choices and flexible responses to their needs.

Before we begin to make provision for those needs we must be clear about why we are doing it: what we want to achieve and why. This means beginning with an understanding of what we value most: what is most important.

There is no single agreed purpose for residential Homes, nor is there a single, simple place for them in the increasingly complicated range of health and social services provision. They meet a lot of varying needs for a wide variety of people. It is therefore not easy to begin to outline the residential worker's task. A start can be made by setting out some statements about the values and principles which are necessary to providing a good quality of life for elderly people.

There is a marked degree of agreement about what these are. The words used may differ slightly but the basic understanding of what is most important – about *why* it is right to do things in a particular way – is the same. *Home Life: A Code of Practice for Residential Care* (Centre for Policy on Ageing, 1984), for instance, says that residents have a fundamental right to self-determination and individuality. Equally, it goes on, they have a right to live in a similar way and circumstances to those which are regarded as normal for people who remain in their own homes. It then lists 'basic rights which should be accorded to all who find themselves in the care of others':

- fulfilment;
- dignity;
- autonomy;
- individuality;
- esteem;
- quality of experience;
- normal opportunities for emotional expression;
- responsible risk-taking and choice.

Some of the principles which have been introduced in the literature on Homes can be regarded as fundamental not so much in the sense that some values are morally good, but rather that particular rights are necessary in an industrialized society if older people are to lead their lives with basic opportunities for achieving satisfaction. And in the end it is whether people have a feeling of satisfaction or well-being which will mark success.

In order to develop these ideas a little further a distinction will be made here between fundamental rights and the operational principles by which they are put into practice.

FUNDAMENTAL RIGHTS

Independence: being in control

One of the most familiar is the right to be independent, often expressed in policy statements as the right of elderly people to live independently in their own homes in the community for as long as possible. This needs to be approached quite carefully. Independence is sometimes used as a description of personality ('this person is fiercely independent') and sometimes as a way of describing material circumstances ('living independently', 'of independent means'). People may be independent in the sense that they manage their physical needs yet not actually *feel* independent. Compare, for example, the position of an elderly woman living in her own home but dependent on neighbours, family and home help to collect her pension, clean the house, empty the commode and light a fire, with that of someone of similar age living in a residential Home but able to dress herself, with no worries about meals, washing-up, getting the laundry done, etc. Each is dependent on others for many things: each may feel either dependent or independent if she feels she retains control over the things in her life that are important to her.

To be able to retain true independence, people must have and maintain an adequate income and a level of health and mobility. It is probably not physical independence alone that is most important but, rather, the feeling of control over one's own life and decisions. It is important to remember, too, that people need others on whom they can depend and to whom they can give in return. The mutual and reciprocal dependence of close and loving relationships is as necessary as the feeling of control that goes with independence. It has been suggested that perhaps the child's most important right is to be a child. Similarly our enthusiasm for the elderly person's right to independence must not blind us to their right to be dependent – to interact with and be supported by others.

In the light of this, it might be better to talk in terms of *interdependence* rather than independence. What is important to elderly people – as to people of any age – is that they should feel needed and useful and that there is a purpose to their life. Involvement and interdependence with others helps to give a feeling of self-esteem.

Respect: being recognized and valued

In some senses many older people living very protected institutional lives but able to dress themselves and move around in wheelchairs may have a more positive self-concept and higher self-esteem (and thereby *feel* more independent) than others living in their own homes but barely surviving, with considerable physical support from others. We must not lose sight of the value of a lifetime of experience and must respect and use that experience in dealing with elderly people. In a Home of 40 people with an average age of around 84 years, there will be approaching 3,500 years of hard-won life experience – to be valued, respected and learned from.

Individuality: being different

Linked to this concept of respect is the importance of treating people as individuals and of recognizing their right to be different. This is especially important in residential Homes where intrusions into privacy are commonplace, quiet corners are rare and the private world of the individual is exposed.

Choice: being free

The concept of quality of life has also been closely linked to the right to choice, sometimes expressed as self-determination. A decrease in choice has frequently been described as a consequence of the ageing process, as the next chapter will illustrate in some detail. As people grow older they tend to experience losses: of family, friends, work roles and relationships, health, income, etc. Each loss brings with it a reduction in the range of choices open to them.

There should be real choices available to older people. If they are to make choices then they must know what is available to them and they may need help in understanding and choosing from among the options. They may also need some help in living with the consequences of some of their decisions! For many elderly residents, choices are few and far between and even the choice of coming into the Home may have been illusory. As one elderly resident put it: 'Yesterday I had a choice of puddings – blancmange, sago, or prunes: that wasn't a choice – that was a dilemma!'

And being responsible

Making choices sometimes exposes people to an element of danger. This raises some interesting and complex issues which are very much a part of the daily work of residential care and which will be considered in detail later. Elderly people have the same rights to decide to choose to do something risky as anyone else, as long as to do so does not put others at risk. They also have the right to expect that residential workers will help them to understand what the risks are so that they can make informed choices.

To summarize, elderly people have a right to be independent but also to interact with and be dependent on others, to be treated with respect for their individuality and unique experience, and to make informed choices amongst a range of real options even if this involves a degree of risk to themselves (and as long as they behave responsibly towards other people) – to decide as far as possible the kind of lives they want for themselves.

OPERATIONAL PRINCIPLES

There is no evidence that I am aware of that these basic values or rights have changed substantially over a long period. It seems likely that most would agree now, as they would have agreed ten or 20 years ago and will continue to agree, that independence, self-determination and respect for individuals should underpin our actions and provision of services. What does tend to change, however, is the way in which we expect to put them into practice.

As a simple example, privacy is now regarded as a key principle for provision of care and most people would now regard a single room as a minimum requirement, except in very special circumstances, in residential Homes. Twenty or 30 years ago this was much less the accepted or usual practice, although privacy was then also an important principle.

With this proviso, that some of the principles of practice by which we seek to meet the basic needs of elderly people shift over time, it is possible to pick out some key principles deriving broadly from the fundamental rights.

The Wagner Report (1988) listed several basic principles which included:

- people should only go into residential care by positive choice;
- no one should have to change their accommodation only to get services which could be provided to them in their own home;
- living in a Home should give a better experience than is available to that person elsewhere;
- the special needs of people from ethnic minority communities should be met;
- the basic human rights of individuals in Homes must be safeguarded;
- people in Homes should have access to community services;
- residents should have access to community facilities and be able to invite family and friends into the Home;
- the value of residential staff needs to be recognized and their contribution enhanced.

To these we can add:

- residents should have a clear statement of the terms and conditions of their residence;
- where residents cannot understand and agree to these, a third party should be available to protect their interests;
- everyone in residential care should have the right to a full assessment of their needs and an opportunity to consider the options available to them.

It will, of course, be possible to develop and break down these points much further; they will be discussed at much more length as the book progresses.

THE WORDS WE USE: A NOTE ON TERMINOLOGY

This book is about providing assistance to elderly people who need some help with the more intimate tasks of everyday living (usually known as personal care) and a sheltered place to live. In the main this means people who live in residential Homes but, in a changing world of health and personal social services provision, it includes a range of other things. There are a lot of forms of special accommodation in which elderly people live and receive help, support or personal care which would not fit easily into the category of residential Home (although most would be thought of as 'home' by those who live there). Some of the problems of terminology and boundaries will be explored in more detail later. Difficulties of definition and administrative boundaries should not be allowed to become a hindrance to flexible and creative thinking about helping elderly people, wherever they live, in a tactful and understanding way.

Before proceeding further, however, it will be useful to consider and define some of the common words:

Elderly: the next chapter will expand on this. Increasing numbers of people reach retirement age. It is particularly important to begin by recognizing that the fact that they do so does not mean that they become any less the unique and different individuals they have always been. It is not appropriate to speak of 'the elderly' as if everyone of a certain age can be described in identical terms. It is also increasingly the case that it is the much older age groups who are likely to be using social services provisions. 'Elderly' has therefore come to refer especially to people over the age of 75 for the purposes of provision of social services.

This book uses the term 'elderly people' for consistency. Other terms have been advocated (elders, elderly citizens, older people, etc.) as being in some sense more respectful. What is really important is not the words we use but rather the respect we feel and demonstrate for the individuality of each person.

Home: this, too, is developed in more detail later, particularly in Chapter 4. The term 'home' will be used to refer to the place people regard as their own personal accommodation space and the domestic needs and expectations associated with this. Where the discussion is about those institutions where large groups of people live together and share the great majority of the accommodation and facilities, the capital letter will be used to show the difference between home and 'Home'. This will become clearer in later discussion of another key word: institution.

17

Care: a word that stands out, if only because of the frequency with which it is used. Caring is a feeling that is experienced by people but it also refers to something done by some people for others. Some of the ways in which the word is used and the meanings given to it will be developed. In the main, it will be used to refer to help given with the personal and intimate tasks of daily life.

Where the gender of an elderly person, worker or other person is not defined by the circumstances described, he or she is referred to throughout the book by the feminine pronoun, since the majority of elderly residents and residential Homes staff are women. Such references should not be taken to imply male or female. The use of the feminine pronoun has been adopted for convenience and to avoid clumsy repetition.

And finally. . . .

The end-product of residential care – in spite of all that will be said about mixed purposes and ambivalence about institutions – is satisfied customers. It is relatively easy to find out whether consumers are satisfied with chocolate dessert: if they want it, they buy it, if they like it, they keep buying it. Finding out whether Homes are successful in ensuring customer satisfaction is more difficult. For now, it is enough to remember that the main measure of whether Homes are 'doing it right' will be whether the residents like what they are getting.

Chapter Two

RESPECTING DIFFERENCES, ACCEPTING SIMILARITIES: ON AGEING AND BEING OLD

This chapter explores some of the ways in which we might try to explain and understand what happens to people as they grow older.

It draws from *gerontology*, which is the study of normal ageing processes. Gerontology developed mainly from the base of work done in North America, although British academics and researchers have done a great deal to refine the basic theoretical propositions in the 1970s and 1980s. It is a discipline which incorporates knowledge and ideas from a number of areas of academic study, especially social policy, psychology, sociology and biology.

It is both the strength and weakness of the study of ageing that it is possible to draw from such a wide base. It is a strength in that there is a depth and richness of resources for knowledge but a weakness because it is extremely difficult to provide a coherent overview or summary of all the issues. It is not the main purpose of this book to provide an introduction to social gerontology. However, some understanding of what ageing means in society generally, as well as for individuals, is necessary before going on to discuss how help can be given most appropriately and effectively.

Gerontology is at a relatively early stage of development. Much of what we understand about ageing, in spite of considerable research effort, is based on imaginative speculation. The picture presented in this chapter assumes that four underlying perspectives need to be taken into account:

1 ageing as a process;
2 old age as a stage or phase of life;

3 the experience of individuals as they get older;
4 the place of elderly people as a group within society.

Much of what has been written about elderly people starts by considering those who find old age a time of problems. 'Old age' is seen as a time of loss, ill health and dependence. We need to be able to step back from this 'snapshot' view of some elderly people at a point in time (although undoubtedly some very elderly people do have difficulties at any particular moment). We must see the impact of ageing processes on all of us in order properly to understand what they mean for each of us.

WHO IS OLD?

The main reason for the growth of interest in ageing and policies for elderly people is quite simply the increase in the numbers and the proportion of older people in our society.

In the last 50 years or so, the numbers of people over 65 in Britain have more than doubled. Those aged 75 and over have increased by almost four times. Fifty years ago one person in 14 was over 65: now the figure is around one in seven. This growth has been particularly marked amongst women. Among the over-75s they outnumber men by two to one.

Between the censuses of 1901 and 1981 the numbers of people aged 65 and over grew from 1.7 million to almost 8 million. This rapid increase has now slowed down. Between 1981 and 2001 it is expected that the over-65s will increase by a little over 12 per cent: in the 20 years from 1961 to 1981 the increase was around one-third.

Life expectancy has increased substantially too. Men and women born in 1910 could expect to live an average of 53 years. Life expectancy is now an average of 75 years. Women can expect to live longer than men: an average of 77.8 years compared to 72.1.

One common way of defining 'old age' has been retirement age. This has been a convenient cut-off point for a number of purposes but hardly reflects the realities that most people experience. To describe anyone over the age of 60 or 65 as old is to include as much as 40 years of remaining life, representing a vast spectrum of different life experience, ability, expectations, etc.

A distinction has begun to be made, therefore, between the

'young old' and the 'old old'. It is those over 75 and especially those over 85 who are most likely to experience reductions in physical, social and economic resources.

Between 1981 and 2001 the younger group, those between 65 and 75 years of age, is likely actually to reduce in absolute numbers.

In the same period, the numbers of those over 75 will grow by a little over 40 per cent, while the numbers of those over 85 will more than double.

Retirement age has itself become more flexible. There has been a growing pattern of early retirement, especially for women. It is noticeable that advertising campaigns increasingly seem to aim at the over-55s for the marketing of certain kinds of leisure, investment and specialist accommodation options, etc.

The simple idea of 'old age' is therefore not so simple. Many people in later middle-age, during their sixties and even seventies, find themselves providing care to older relatives, especially parents. It is probably more appropriate to think of the concept of 'the elderly' as applying to people over the age of 75 or even older. This is the group that continues to grow as a proportion of the population as a whole and even more markedly as a proportion of those over retirement age. They are also the people who are more likely to make heavier demands on Health and Social Services provision.

But it is not particularly productive to dwell on the concept of old age. It is a description of people who have little in common but the length of time they have all been alive. It is more helpful to think about the process of ageing through time. There are some key words which can be used to develop a consideration of some of the most important aspects of that process. They include: loss, change, separation, adaptation, exchange and activity. These are all elements of the *social process* of ageing.

A SOCIAL PROCESS

Time and transition

One way of viewing ageing is to see it as a continuous process of change and development through time. This has sometimes been called the life-cycle. This idea of a cycle of life has usually been applied to the process of reproduction in animals – birth, growth, reproduction and death. The human life-span has increasingly been extended beyond the age of reproduction (although it is not so much that people are living longer: rather, more people are living to the maximum life-span). This has led some writers to suggest that the term 'life-path' (or 'life-course') might be a more appropriate description.

The life-path, or progress through life, has a series of recogniz-able phases or stages which apply to most, but not necessarily all, people. At the most basic these include childhood, young adult-hood, middle-age and old age. There are more complicated ways of listing these stages in relation, for example, to the tasks to be accomplished at various ages, such as growing up, leaving home, marriage, having children, finding a successful work role, caring for children and ageing parents, retirement, etc. These are considered again later in the chapter, in the discussion of success-ful ageing.

A helpful approach which provides a bridge between attempts to describe the needs of all older people over a certain age as well as the experiences of each individual who reaches that age has been called the biographical approach. This stresses the unique-ness of each person's own life story or personal history. It is argued that ageing can be understood as an individual experience of life, which can be set in the context of experiences common to others of the same age but which will have its own distinct reality and meaning.

It is, however, probably most useful to think of ageing as not just one single process but as a collection of processes. Each person experiences various social, psychological, emotional and intel-lectual change processes as life progresses. There are some things which happen to most people during that general process but it is difficult to make definite statements about what is 'normal' at any particular stage of life. People may be similar but they are all different!

Loss and deprivation

Ageing has frequently been described as a time of loss. As people grow older they begin to lose some of their social roles: the tasks they perform in society, with all the associated expectations they and others have of them.

Perhaps the most significant role losses are associated with employment. Retirement from work brings with it a range of changes for both men and women which have a major impact on their lives. There are, of course, many other role losses and changes, but retirement is particularly significant because of its association with loss of money and other material resources.

Sociological explanations of ageing experiences fall broadly into two groups. Some describe elderly people as victims of an unequal industrial society. Others have been more concerned with the social roles which people play or are expected to play, considering the extent to which people adjust to society's expectations or to which they remain aloof or detached from them.

Elderly people, seen as victims, are presented as a direct burden within the capitalist state, making no contribution to either capital wealth or the mode of production. In this sense the problems encountered with ageing are problems of oppression and material deprivation.

The extent to which this is so for individuals is likely to be related to the status and income people have achieved before retirement. Those with higher status and income are more likely to continue to maintain a materially better life-style. Patterns of family life vary similarly. Where people have had higher occupational status and retain a higher income in later life, the direction of help in the family is more likely to be from parent to child than in families where the parent's occupational status and income are lower.

Women have been described as being particularly vulnerable. It has been argued, for instance, that such discussions of occupational status and social class have very little relevance to women because of their unequal status both in the labour market and in the home.

Similarly, attention has been drawn to the position of elderly people from black and other ethnic minority groups. People who have grown old in Britain but who may still feel themselves to be strangers are more likely than the indigenous population to be living in conditions of loneliness, sickness, fear and deprivation. They experience particular powerlessness: they have greater difficulty in getting access to services, treatment and resources because of differences in language, culture, skin colour or religious belief, which compound any problems of ageing.

Giving and receiving

The relative imbalance of power between older and younger people is particularly important in understanding the ageing experience. The exchange of goods, gifts and services is one way in which bonds of trust and mutual support are developed in society. It leads to gratitude, obligation and the development of relationships. There is, however, an expectation of reciprocity: that one party will respond to another in exchange for what is given or received. If there is no reciprocity then the giver tends to gain power or control over the receiver: this is the foundation of dependence.

It has been argued that elderly people in industrialized society have little power and therefore devalue themselves and are devalued. This leads to negative stereotyping: they may be excluded from the chance to work and earn money, have restricted social opportunities and lose social roles.

This view emphasizes the decreasing resources and therefore loss of power experienced with ageing. Older people are said to be increasingly weak in their social exchanges with younger people. This growing imbalance in social interaction forces elderly people to exchange compliance with the wishes of younger people in return for continued support and resources. The older person is in a 'can't win' situation. Access to power and resources declines with age, placing the elderly person in a position of weakness when negotiating. At the same time some resources have to be exchanged for less than they would be if held by a younger person: the things older people have to offer are often not valued as highly.

This is an important element of care in a residential Home. The attitudes of carers and of residents are likely to be influenced by the extent to which the relationship is seen as reciprocal (the resident pays for services received) or based on power (one party – usually the carer – is seen to be more powerful).

Passivity and activity

One of the earliest and most influential sociological propositions about ageing has been known as 'disengagement theory'. In its original form this proposed that the social process of ageing is characterized by a gradual reduction in social interaction for the ageing individual, who was held to need less involvement. There were said to be three elements of withdrawal: a loss of social roles or activities, a reduction in social contacts and a reduced commitment to social norms and values. As people grow older, it was suggested, society demands less of them and this is acceptable and even necessary to them. In this sense, a 'satisfying old age' actually requires reduced activity and involvement.

This view is now rarely defended in its original form. More recent considerations of the disengagement approach have taken a less extreme view, arguing simply that it is possible but not essential to be uninvolved or segregated from important activities and contacts and yet still lead a satisfying old age.

In some contrast, what has become known as the 'activity theory' of ageing proposes that the levels of an individual's satisfaction with life will be directly related to the amount of social activity. There is, of course an important distinction between physical activity and social activity in this context. It has also been argued that health and physical well-being are related to the maintenance of exercise and general physical activity.

Disengagement and activity explanations have often been presented as opposing views, although they are concerned with rather different issues. One important factor seems to be the personality dimension: the kind of person she is and the way she has learned to view the world in general is likely to be a major influence on whether an individual sees an active or a quiet life as desirable.

The problem of accepting a disengagement view of the world is that, if it is taken literally, we would expect elderly people to sit passively and watch the world go by (or, at the extreme, not even bother to watch). The effect of such a view would be to limit services to the provision of the minimum necessary to create a warm, safe environment. There is ample evidence that many people at all ages – whether they be 65, 85 or 95 – do choose active involvement in social roles and relationships.

Involvement and adjustment

The disadvantage of all such theories and approaches is that they are very generalized. They assume that there is a large degree of similarity about people over a similar age. The evidence that people can be viewed in such common or homogeneous terms is very dubious. There may be very broad social pressures which create some similarities between people in age groups. But the most important influences on individual satisfaction in old age are probably health, lack of disease or illness and personality factors.

There is no doubt that many retired people have found old age a time of relative poverty and lack of material possessions. On the other hand, it is clear that most elderly people are involved or integrated into their local communities by the services they provide to others, by their relationships with family and friends and by the services they receive in return.

However, a substantial minority of elderly people are isolated from family and friends (although this depends on many things: age, gender, social class, marital status, etc.). What seems to be important is probably not the objective facts of integration or involvement but the way people *feel* about what they are able to do. If they regard their social contacts and activities as appropriate, they are more likely to feel satisfied with life, whatever the real level of contacts looks like to the outside observer. In other words, it is how they feel about what is happening in their lives that is most important.

Social processes: a summary

Some key elements can be drawn for emphasis from this brief review:

1 Elderly people as a group are relatively less well-off in a material sense than younger people, although wealth is unequally and variably distributed amongst them.
2 In consequence, they are relatively less powerful and as a group are more likely to be dependent on others for the resources they need.
3 Satisfaction with life may, for some people, be related to a withdrawal from or reduction in social activities. For others it

may be related to maintaining or changing social activities. Particularly important is the way an individual subjectively perceives her level of involvement and activity: whether she feels it is what she wants.

4 In order to understand elderly people it is essential to recognize their unique individuality. A helpful way of making a start on this is to consider, with them, their personal life history. This must be set in the light of the common experiences of all elderly people and the pressures which society as a whole creates for them.

The pattern that tends to emerge suggests that ageing is a social process of gradually lessening involvement for most (but not all) people. Undoubtedly, older people as a whole do remain integrated into society and continue to get satisfaction from taking part in family and social activities and relationships. For a minority of people rather more roles may be lost for a variety of reasons – personal choice, failing health, bereavement, or reduced material resources. Some may choose to 'disengage': it is those who are 'compulsorily' deprived of active roles and relationships who are most likely to experience ageing in problem terms.

Basically, understanding ageing as a social phenomenon means understanding the balance of three things:

- the fact that social structures and attitudes do create common expectations which affect all older people;
- the common life experiences of people in the same age group;
- the differences between individuals (especially personality and life experiences).

A PHYSICAL PROCESS

Ageing is also a physical process with readily recognizable, central features. There is, however, little agreement on what causes the body to age.

There have been some engaging explanations. A Russian biologist, for instance, proposed at the turn of the century that the noxious bacteria in the digestive system produce putrefaction, leading to ageing effects. His solution was to eat yoghurt (Metchnikoff, quoted in Birren 1986). It is also claimed that in ancient

Hindustan, 'persons suffering from senile debility were given the testicles of a tiger to eat' (Schmidt 1931). Given the problems of administering and, not least, of obtaining this prescription, it is perhaps fortunate that approaches are now slightly more sophisticated!

The search for immortality or at least an extended and active life, has a long history. It was not until the twentieth century that very old people became more numerous. There have always been some people living into old age, but the likelihood of a seventh and eighth decade has only recently become a reality for the majority.

Some understanding of the normal processes of ageing – those things which happen to most people as they grow older – is necessary to begin to disentangle the physical changes which can be regarded as abnormal or unusual: the pathological changes of illness and disease. Some of the most common features of ageing seem to be changes in the arteries, changes in the body's immune system leading to a reduced resistance to infection, and loss of brain cells.

A variety of explanations have been offered for these ageing effects. These include the accumulation of a series of biological damages caused by illnesses and general 'wear and tear' over the years; and a possible in-built genetic predisposition or 'programming' for 'built-in obsolescence'.

The rate at which changes occur is not uniform and is affected by both the personality characteristics of the individual and by the environment. Some people survive by fighting and thrive on struggle and hard work, but often age at no faster or slower rate than others who live a more protected and dependent existence. The best guess seems to be that the body grows older in response to an inherited set of characteristics which are influenced by the environment, opportunities and pressures experienced by each individual.

Some of the most common age-related changes are:

Many people undergo changes in posture and a slight decline in stature is usual. Elderly people are characteristically shorter in the trunk of the body with comparatively long arms and legs: the opposite of the pattern of growth in the young child. Height is lost, partly as a result of changes in the discs of the spine but also because of a tendency to bend or stoop, especially at the knees or hips.

The skin of the older person becomes thinner and wrinkled. Creasing of the skin, due to loss of fat around the eyes and the effects of the muscles of expression leads to wrinkling of the face and a typically sunken appearance of the eyes. Loss of the fatty layer below the skin contributes to wrinkling and general loss of elasticity of the skin results in sagging.

The hair goes grey and there is often a loss of hair both on the head and elsewhere on the body as the follicles become fewer. Muscle strength diminishes with age and bones become weaker through loss of calcium. Blood pressure often rises; blood flow may be restricted because of the depositing of fat on the artery walls (atherosclerosis) and when the walls become thicker or less resilient (arterio-sclerosis).

There are changes in the senses. In the eye, presbyopia (a form of long-sightedness) develops, typically from the mid-forties onwards. Changes in hearing develop at a similar age with a gradually increasing difficulty in receiving higher frequencies. Most people are able to compensate for these changes for many years, but elderly people usually have some degree of hearing loss. They sometimes have difficulty in picking out conversations between people: the so-called 'cocktail-party' effect where it is difficult for them to separate out different sounds. The senses of smell and taste are also likely to become less acute with age, although often not until much later in life. The quality of sleep may also decline as sleep patterns change: the duration and depth of sleep may be affected.

As these and other changes accumulate, the elderly person is less likely to be able to respond effectively to the stresses of physical demands. The longer a person lives, the more likely she is to acquire a collection of illnesses and diseases. In turn, these contribute to increasing the pressures on the ageing body.

AN INTELLECTUAL PROCESS

The processes of change in intellectual ability – the ability to think, reason, analyse and understand – which occur during ageing are also complex. In spite of considerable research in the last 30 years, there is much that is still poorly understood, unclear or unexplained.

The ability to think creatively has been said to peak quite early in life. Mathematical and scientific thinkers are said to do most of their best work in the first three of four decades of their lives. Most successful creative writers tend to write their best work before they are 40. Yet there are examples of people who have produced outstanding creative contributions to science and literature much later in life.

It is certainly possible to 'teach old dogs new tricks'. There is good evidence that many elderly people are perfectly able to take up new activities, to learn complex tasks, and to acquire an understanding of elaborate concepts. Some research has suggested that older people are likely to be slower to learn and more cautious in new situations than younger people. Yet some elderly people are much more able than most younger people: on various tests they can learn more quickly and can perform more successfully.

Interpreting the evidence is difficult. Some of the factors which influence the intellectual performance of elderly people may be:

1 Their health: some of the reported slowness or relative inefficiency of older people on psychological laboratory testing may be explained by the limitations imposed by illness or discomfort.

2 Their motivation: there is some evidence that the performance of elderly people on tests of intellectual ability is related to the potential rewards. Where the potential pay-offs are greater, their ability to perform increases and their reported caution about decision making reduces.

3 Their attitude to ageing: there are strong stereotypes in society, as has already been established. If elderly people have learned these and have accepted them, they may under-perform because they have low expectations.

4 Their opportunities: skills deteriorate and if there is no chance to practise, to develop and maintain skills, then the

ability to handle concepts and decisions may be reduced.
5 The effects of chronic (or acute) brain changes.

These factors are very important from the point of view of providing good residential care. The maintenance of intellectual ability is likely to be dependent on, or at least aided by, good health and well-being, encouragement and motivation, positive attitudes and a stimulating environment. It also seems reasonable to assume that a positive, encouraging and stimulating mental, social and physical environment is likely to lead to feelings of satisfaction and contentment, as well as improved skills and abilities.

BEING A PROBLEM AND HAVING PROBLEMS

'Normal' and 'not-normal'

So far this discussion has concentrated on ageing as a collection of normal processes: 'normal' in the sense that they are experienced by most people as they grow older in our society. At any point in time some elderly people experience substantial problems and some are seen by society as 'a problem'.

The danger of discussing the problems of old age is that we may tend to emphasize the negatives of the ageist view criticized earlier. We must not lose sight of the overall view of ageing as a process.

But what are the problems and whose problems are they?

It was earlier shown that there are many more elderly people than there used to be. There is a 'problem of old age' in the sense that there are increasing numbers relative to the number of people available to provide care and support. But the development of a policy for an ageing population is much more complicated than just counting the numbers. It means making some fundamental decisions about the place of elderly people in society.

Ageing has not been seen consistently as a problem by politicians and policy makers. There is a real sense in which the increase in survival represents a triumph of improved health and social wellbeing. Policies are needed which will capitalize on this triumph by developing varied opportunities for a new leisured group.

Neither has ageing always been seen as the same kind of problem. One view, for example, sees ageing as problematic because it brings suffering and costs for elderly people: policies need to focus on problem-solving for individuals to reduce the discomforts of old age. Another view presents the main problem as that which arises for society as a whole from increasing numbers of unproductive, burdensome elderly people. Policies in this sense are focused on reducing the costs to the community as a whole.

Throughout the life process individuals are likely to encounter events and opportunities which may lead to problems. People are affected differently by similar events. As a simple example, we know that some people look forward to retirement as a time when they will be able to do all the things they never had time for before. Others dread it as a cutting-off of the relationships and other rewards they get from work. After retirement, the reactions are equally varied and often not at all what people expected.

In spite of these general qualifications, there are some features of age which are likely to cause particular difficulty. These include poverty, mental health changes and physical disability. A brief review of some of the more common issues follows, but, before proceeding, two points should be stressed:

1 We should not overreact to the difficulties experienced by *some* elderly people and make generalized assumptions that *all* elderly people have similar problems. Nevertheless, although only a minority of elderly people have problems at any time, an increasing number can expect to have problems and to use health and personal social services resources at some stage in their lives: usually as they reach greater age.
2 The basic values that were outlined earlier – independence, self-determination, choice, quality of life, etc. – remain constant as basic assumptions of this discussion. What does tend to change, however, is what we are willing to regard – and can afford to regard – as 'adequate' provision to meet needs. Policy objectives may be broadly consistent but actual operational practice will shift over time. Not least this is necessary as new issues are identified and treatments or solutions developed (e.g. hypothermia; physical abuse of elderly people; new housing options).

32

Family strain and the needs of carers

It is important to begin with a recognition of how the problems of elderly people can affect the lives of those around them. Many of the difficulties are of families or couples (e.g. retirement; reduced income; relationship changes). Many take place in, or have a very direct effect on, families. Even the problems of elderly people living alone are likely to have direct implications for those who care for them.

One adult in seven in Great Britain provides informal care and one household in five contains a carer. The peak age for caring is 45 to 64: a fifth of adults in this age range provide informal care. Women are a little more likely than men to be carers, but since there are more women than men in the total population the actual number of women is much higher. About half of carers have dependants over 75 years of age. The most common circumstance is carers looking after parents living outside their own household. Nearly two-thirds of carers carry the main responsibility (Green 1988)

Writing about caring for her mother, who had suffered a severe stroke, Patricia Slack comments on the mixture of feelings:

> We learnt how to manage as we went along. Useful inform-ation was difficult to find . . . I found that carers' accounts of the emotions surrounding their experiences helped me to grapple with the cauldron of love, remorse, anger, fear, hatred and violence which boiled inside me.
>
> (Slack and Mulville 1987: viii)

She adds:

> Caring for a severely disabled relative is demanding and exhausting . . . We hear little about the rewards. My mother showed Frank and me a new depth and breadth of love for each other. Her tragedy formed the basis for the most enrich-ing emotional experience of our lives.
>
> (ibid.: ix)

Others have described the strains which can develop as tasks taken on willingly and from a sense of love or duty become a burden. Ruth Cowling's story is included in a collection of experiences of carers (Briggs and Oliver 1985). She was caring for her mother and assisting her blind husband. She says:

> Looking back, I see that what began as a pleasant duty became an intolerable burden and I was not able to convince those who had it within their power to help me that I really had reached the point where I could no longer cope single-handed. . . Our society expects a woman to care for her dependant twenty-four hours a day, seven days a week, for fifty weeks in every fifty-two. I believe that our society is expecting too much of the carer.
>
> (Briggs and Oliver 1985: 6)

In the same collection, Pat Waterman writes of the experience of caring for her mother and an elderly aunt following the death of her husband. She illustrates the particular frustrations of caring for a confused person:

> Few people can understand the sense of desperation, left alone for long periods with a confused elderly person, unless they have done it themselves. It makes you do and say cruel things, even though you love the person . . What I want for Mum is a relatively easy time of it for what there is left, because I can't bear to see her suffer, and before it gets too bad, an easy, merciful way out – peacefully at home, I hope, with me holding her hand.
>
> (ibid.: 64–5)

Strain develops in many areas of the life of the family or carer. The demands of providing care may intrude into work, leisure, marriage and care of children. The stress may show in the deteriorating health of the carer and in emotional and psychological distress.

Often, children of ageing parents find the burden of care descending on them when they are in their fifties or sixties. This is at a time when they may have expected to be able to relax and start to develop leisure and hobbies after child-care responsibilities begin to reduce. This may lead to mixed feelings of duty and responsibility yet resentment with consequent ambivalence and frustration. Many, of course, take on helping relatives or friends willingly and find pleasure in doing so. The increasing burden as problems increase becomes intolerable for some.

Work and money

There is a trend in Britain towards early retirement. There are few men or women who now remain economically active beyond the normal retirement age. This is related to changing attitudes to work and leisure and probably also to changing employment and unemployment patterns. When there is a surplus of labour in the employment market the tendency is to look to retirement as a means of reducing that surplus.

The way life is experienced in the early years after retirement depends on several factors. Continuing good health and income level are clearly essential to the enjoyment of an active life. Retirement brings loss of interaction with workmates and other contacts but may offer new opportunities for greater involvement with family and friends. Social class factors are influential. Social and geographical mobility are linked and families may be widely scattered.

Most people do not miss work after retirement. Whether they are able to put things they enjoy in the place of work, however, depends on various things: interest and motivation, whether they have always had an active interest in hobbies and leisure, and whether they can afford to pay.

Elderly people as a group are relatively poor. Just over one in four people over retirement age have incomes at or below the usually quoted poverty line (the point at which they require state support in addition to the basic retirement pension). Their poverty is particularly related to two things: they have little access to ways of increasing their income by working; and the assets they do have are likely to be reducing in value (through, for example, deterioration in the condition of housing or inflation).

Women have additional difficulties. If unmarried, their income is likely to have been lower and their reserves will be smaller. Occupational pensions may have been linked to husbands and widows are often left with suddenly reduced incomes. Women are also likely to live to greater age than men. They are therefore more likely to see their resources dwindle for all these reasons. The older both men and women grow, the less likely they are to have an income sufficient for their needs.

A place to live

Most elderly people are living in the community. Only about 3 per cent of those over 65 are in residential care, although this proportion increases markedly with greater age.

The proportion of owner-occupiers and Council tenants among two-person households where both the occupants are over 65 is similar to that in the general population. But where there is an elderly householder alone, he or she is much more likely to be a Council or private tenant.

Elderly people living alone, especially those over the age of 75, have the worst housing conditions. Almost three times as many as in the general population had no bath or inside WC at the 1981 census. They are also more likely to be in housing without central heating. They face problems of maintaining older housing where they are owner-occupiers and problems of releasing capital which is tied up in the housing, although a variety of schemes now exist to assist with this.

Friends, neighbours and companionship

About half of women over 65 live alone, compared to about one in five men. The likelihood of living alone is greatest among the very elderly; this is especially so for women.

Being alone is not necessarily an unpleasant experience: many people of all ages choose to be alone. But living alone is associated with isolation from social contacts and isolation is in turn linked with the feeling of loneliness.

Research consistently shows the importance of family, friends and good neighbours to elderly people. Where they feel they have good and supportive contacts, elderly people are more likely to say they are happy, contented or satisfied.

Not all elderly people experience living alone but the longer they live the greater becomes the chance that they will live alone (although people over 80, especially women, are more likely than younger people to be living with family other than a spouse). The likelihood of isolation and therefore of loneliness also grows with age.

Bereavement and death

Elderly people are, of course, nearer to death. Some will view the prospect with anxiety, fear or confusion; others regard it in a matter-of-fact way. Attitudes amongst people vary and the feelings of individuals about what death means to them fluctuate over time.

Usually, what people seem to fear is not death itself but the pain which they expect may attend the process of dying. People who are in good health and who express a spiritual trust or religious faith are less likely to express fears of dying.

Unfortunately, some elderly people are exposed to dying in an unpleasant manner, perhaps in pain, distress or alone. In the period before death there is evidence of a good deal of unreported illness amongst elderly people and of distressing symptoms (such as unpleasant smells, loss of bladder control) which could be relieved with medical treatment, but for which no one has been consulted.

Elderly people are likely to experience the loss of close family and friends: the older they become, the more likely this is. They are therefore more likely to experience bereavement and grief which in turn may contribute to increased strain on mental and physical health.

Ill health and disability

Some of the changes which affect the human body with age have already been described. These changes affect the general level of physical functioning.

The incidence of illness and associated disability increases with age. Much of this is unidentified in the sense that elderly people do not present many of their symptoms to doctors for diagnosis. Studies of illness amongst elderly people have consistently found considerable levels of illness, previously undiagnosed.

It would not be appropriate to attempt a detailed discussion here but some elements are worthy of special note.

1 Failure to thrive

This is an expression that has been used to describe the common complaint of elderly people that they cannot 'perform' as normal.

This is often put down to 'just old age' but calls for a full medical assessment to establish cause and effect and potential treatments.

2 Accidents and falls

Falls are common amongst elderly people and may have a number of causes. They are important as they may be symptomatic of other problems and because of their potential to lead to other problems (a long wait for help, hospitalization, loss of confidence, etc.). Accidents are a major cause of death and disablement in both men and women over the age of 65.

3 Hypothermia

Exposure to cold is the main cause of hypothermia (a severe drop in body temperature) but this may be related to existing physical problems. There are often problems of the body's ability to regulate its own warmth which can in turn be related to other disease or illness processes.

4 Disability

Disability is actually about the relationship between a person and her environment. It is related to illness, disease and impairment and the things that these prevent an individual from doing. The loss of the use of a leg, for instance, is an impairment which leads to the disability of being unable to climb stairs and the handicap of not being able to sleep upstairs like others do, without special equipment or help. It is therefore not so much 'what is wrong' with people that matters but, rather, what they would like to do but are unable to do.

A survey carried out in 1985 and 1986 estimated that there were just over 6 million adults with one or more disabilities in Great Britain. Around 400,000 of these lived in some kind of communal establishment. Many disabilities are caused by impairments that arise during ageing. The survey found that the overall rate of disability rises with age, slowly at first, accelerating after 50 and rising very steeply after 70. About 70 per cent of disabled adults were 60 or over and nearly half were 70 or over.

Among the most severely disabled, very elderly people predominate. Severe disability rises steeply from the age of 70 and especially so after 80. Sixty-four per cent of adults with the most severe disabilities were over 70 and 41 per cent were 80 or over.

There were more elderly women than men with a disability, both because there are higher numbers of women in this age group and also because women over 75 are more likely to be disabled than men of the same age (Martin *et al.* 1985)

Disability is associated with a loss of mobility: the ability to get about without restriction. This is also linked to income and access to car transport. The relationship between health, disability and mobility is close and each contributes to a reduction in opportunity and therefore in quality of life.

Mental disorder

Forms of dementia make up by far the greatest proportion of mental disorder amongst elderly people. Estimates of the extent of mental disorder amongst the elderly population are uncertain but it seems likely that around one in ten up to the age of 80 and around one in five of those over 80 have severe or moderate dementia. At least one-fifth of people over 65 are said to show some evidence of a serious mental disorder at any one time.

Again, it would not be appropriate to give a detailed description or exploration of the mental disorders that affect elderly people. This is, however, of major significance to the lives and work of people in residential Homes and some introductory discussion is necessary to the subsequent consideration of helping people in Homes. The following are some of the principal disorders:

1 Depression

There is a substantial amount of depressive illness amongst elderly people living in Homes. Often, this is unrecognized. Physical ill health, loss and bereavement increase the likelihood of depression. Sometimes, a depressed person will present symptoms similar to those of someone suffering from dementia: impaired awareness, memory changes and self-neglect.

It is important for residential workers to be aware of the likelihood of depression amongst residents and the chance that it may lead to behaviour very similar to that of people with dementia.

2 Confusional illness

Elderly people may behave in a confused way for many reasons.

Proper assessment and diagnosis are essential and must be carried out by a psychiatrist.

Sometimes, confusional illness is acute and is related to underlying physical illness. It may be caused by infection, stroke, the toxic effects of alcohol or drugs or traumatic illness.

Chronic conditions leading to a set of confused behaviours are known as dementias, sometimes as 'chronic brain failure'. Senile dementia (also called 'dementia of the Alzheimer's type') has a relatively slow onset and the sufferer may live for as long as ten years or so with a pattern of increasing speech and communication difficulty, memory impairment and loss of awareness. Arteriosclerotic or multi-infarct dementia produces similar behavioural changes and the two conditions may often be found together.

The set of symptoms associated with brain failure or dementia (remembering that depression may lead to similar symptoms in some cases) includes:

• memory loss, forgetfulness;
• loss of awareness of place;
• reduced attention span, impaired judgement;
• restlessness, anxiety;
• fixed ideas, suspicion;
• seeing and hearing things that are not there;
• confused memories.

These lead to a variety of problems, including:

• self-neglect;
• accidents in the home;
• wandering;
• stress on carers.

People with dementia are also more likely to experience physical illness.

Some of these issues will be developed in more detail in the later discussion of helping people suffering from dementia in Homes.

A COLLECTION OF PROBLEMS: RISK AND AGEING

This brief review has by no means covered all the potential difficulties that attend the ageing process. Most people can expect to come across some things that they will find a problem, regardless of age. Some elderly people collect more than their fair share of problems and need help; others have particularly serious difficulties which they cannot deal with alone; and others are unable to cope because of the sudden and unexpected onset of difficulties, such as bereavement or stroke or other crisis illness.

Chronological age – the time someone has been alive – is actually less important in determining whether they are at risk of finding old age a time of problems than is their health and income. Whether they can develop leisure activities in retirement, for instance, depends largely on whether they have the energy and money to enjoy it. Similarly, the suitability of housing is likely to depend on whether they can afford the upkeep and continue to manage the stairs, bath or kitchen without help.

It is not very helpful to think about one problem separately from all the others which are linked to it. If someone is short of money then they may not be eating properly or keeping warm and they certainly will not be keeping up social contacts. These factors in turn will contribute to ill health, isolation, loneliness and general failure to thrive. The result is a downward spiral of gradually increasing need.

It is the collecting together of a set of problems which is most likely to lead to need for health and personal social service help. This is especially likely amongst 'old elderly' people: the over-75s and, even more, the over-85s. It is this group who are most likely to find their way into residential Homes. Very elderly people are most at risk of accumulated problems or crisis breakdown.

Two final points should again be stressed:

1 Women are more likely to experience old age as a time of difficulty. They have a greater chance of living in poverty than men and, because they are more likely to live into very old age, they have a greater likelihood of encountering severe disability.
2 Elderly people from black and other ethnic minority groups may also experience ageing in particularly problematic ways. They are more likely to be living in areas of high deprivation, may have moved more frequently and have lower income and savings. On top of all this, they face problems of discrimination and prejudice.

SATISFACTION AND SUCCESS: WHAT IS A 'GOOD OLD AGE'?

What will be regarded as a good and successful old age will depend on how we view the world in general. It will probably also depend on how old we are and where we stand when we view it!

From a broad policy standpoint, a good old age may be found in a society which has a balance of the production of wealth through labour and the consumption of wealth by those who are dependent. In other words, where there is a balance of people of working age with children and elderly people.

From the point of view of the individual elderly person, satisfaction and success may be measured by a range of subjective factors. There is, of course, a world of difference between the wishes and needs of a recently retired couple in their early-sixties, with a close family, their own home, good health and substantial income and savings, and those of a widowed woman of 85 with arthritis, the beginnings of dementia, a rented, terraced house and a son living in Australia!

In all of these situations, however, there are some words and concepts which will have relevance and importance in explaining their situation: health, well-being, welfare, adjustment, etc. These can usefully be considered in more detail.

Health and well-being

Complete health is not just about the absence of illness or disease, but is a sense of overall well-being that comes from a feeling of physical, emotional and social security. There is, of course, a close relationship between illness and physical health. Someone who is generally healthy will be able to cope with and recover from a bout of illness. A more generally frail elderly person is less likely to be able to resist and make a full recovery.

But old age must not be regarded as a state of ill health. There is a slow and symptomless process of biological ageing, as described earlier. The rate at which changes take place during ageing varies from one person to the next. Some of the ageing changes help to make elderly people more vulnerable to illness: but that does not mean old age is an illness. Most of the research about illness and elderly people has looked at how ill they are, rather than how well they are. As noted earlier, there is extensive unreported illness among elderly people who often regard illness as 'just old age'.

Whether people think of themselves as healthy or not depends on a lot of things. Most elderly people say they are in good health for their age: for some, however, the bottle has always been half-empty, for others it is half-full! People may take an optimistic or pessimistic view of the world and this will influence their attitude to their own health. Each person has a view of herself and what she can do. Ageing brings changes to physical abilities from middle-age onwards. Most people get the chance to adjust slowly to these but, for some, crisis illness such as a stroke can call for sudden and, in every sense, painful reassessment.

There is, therefore, a close link between health, physical abilities and self-esteem. Health changes for some elderly people mean a process of learning to be dependent on others: often on children. This can mean a frustrating and difficult adjustment in the nature of long-standing relationships.

Health and well-being are closely related because they are about 'feeling good': a key element in a satisfying old age.

Welfare

In one sense, welfare means much the same as well-being: being in a satisfactory state, enjoying life and being healthy. In a more specific sense, promoting the welfare of elderly people has been used to refer to social policies and social services designed to ensure that individuals do not suffer in old age.

In this second sense, it is helpful to think about two elements:

1 Welfare policies designed to make sure that all elderly people lead a good life: maintaining at least a minimum income, developing specialist housing, etc. These tend to develop around a very general view of a 'good old age'.
2 Welfare services aimed at helping elderly people in difficulty: including home care/home help services, night-sitter services, residential Homes, etc. These tend to be based on limited resources stretched thinly to provide for a lot of people, although there are trends towards a more intensive use of some services for a smaller number in greater need. The focus

is mainly on the minimum that must be done to prevent serious mishap. They are, therefore, mainly about preventing a 'bad old age' more than about creating a 'good old age'.

Adaptation

People grow old in the same way as they have grown up: in their own unique and individual way and in response to their experiences of the environment and relationships they encounter. Research confirms that attitudes to such things as welfare benefits, as well as to their health, are influenced by their subjective view of the world. It is what people regard as normal, what they expect of the world, that governs how they view what happens to them.

If we follow this line too closely, however, we place the responsibility for 'being able to cope', or to 'adapt' or to grow old successfully very much on the individual. Whether or not they lead a good old age becomes dependent on whether they are willing and able to see it that way. Clearly, this is not the whole story.

Many of the pressures on elderly people are outside their control. A successful old age is therefore likely to be a complex of things based around the central theme of the relationship between what a person *wants* for herself and what actually happens to her. This can be thought of as the interrelationship of the inner and outer worlds of the individual.

Perhaps the most positive view is to think of each individual as consciously self-determining in contributing to defining and developing her own world. Some things cannot be changed and we have to learn to live with them. But we can each play some part in 'managing' our environment and in learning to 'manage' within it.

Self and others

The importance of income and health have so far been stressed. Also of central importance is the value of personal relationships.

Some of the rewards of relationships are based on the satisfaction of being involved with, and doing things for, others: on reciprocity in contact with others. Value is placed on social acceptance, concern for others and generally being welcomed by, seen as positive by, and having a positive impact on, others.

Other rewards are essentially self-orientated: they are about what can be got out of contact with others. Such things as self-expression, leisure and activity are important.

Most relationships are based on reciprocity: on give and take. Relationships involve family ties, affection, sexual expression, friendship, etc., and people expect to put something in and get something back. Most elderly people are closely bound into family and community by the things they do for others and have done for them in return.

For most, a satisfying, 'good old age' will be tied up with reciprocal relationships. They need to feel a part of family and friendship ties. Some are more inclined to give than take but the general principle seems to hold good: elderly people need to do and to be done to in return.

Successful ageing and life tasks

How will we recognize successful ageing when we see it?

It is probably a combination of a long life (survival), together with good health, lack of disability and happiness (a feeling of satisfaction and contentment). Happiness is in the eye of the beholder: different people want different things and we must listen to each individual to learn what each wants.

Some writers have stressed the importance of 'life tasks' in understanding ageing. They tend to draw from developmental psychology and some basic propositions are important:

• people continue to grow and change throughout life;
• adulthood can be seen as a progress through a sequence of developments.

This offers a way of thinking about what is happening in people's lives and whether they are on or off course through time. The assumption that adulthood is an orderly progression is, however, a dubious one. For many people, it is disorganized and haphazard with little clear direction.

A useful way of thinking about this is that of Erikson (1964), who emphasizes life tasks and proposes that there are eight stages to be achieved or worked through in the development of the self (or 'ego'). These progress from an initial stage of trust versus mistrust, in which the infant has to learn to accept the behaviour of and separation from his parents, through to a final stage of integration or despair. This final stage or task is mainly about an acceptance of an order and meaning in the individual's total life: to accept all that has gone before as necessary and meaningful. This is said to provide a safe base from which to view the inevitability of death.

The problem with such a view is that at each life stage the principal task has to be achieved before the individual can proceed to the next stage. Many do not lead the kind of orderly and 'ordinary' life that enables such a standard progression. The approach does, however, offer an interesting way of thinking about adjustment to ageing.

In the end, satisfaction and adaptation have to be seen in the context of the social environment as well as in relation to the subjective experience of the individual. People may have made adaptations to their circumstances without necessarily being 'well adjusted': learning to live with something is not necessarily the same as making a good adjustment. The fact that people tolerate their situation does not mean that they find it acceptable or that it is fair that they should have to tolerate it.

AGEING AND OLD AGE: KEY ISSUES

There are a small number of points which are central to our understanding of ageing and old age:

1 Ageing is best understood as a collection of social, physical and intellectual processes.
2 Old age is a chronologically defined time of life: there is a group of people over retirement age who have mainly their age in common. Society as a whole has attitudes to them which they in turn share about themselves. These influence their behaviour and the social policies which are developed for them.
3 The individual experience of old age is strongly influenced by the subjective views of each person: it is how people feel about what happens to them that is important.
4 As people grow older, they may encounter a number of problems: reduced income, inadequate housing, loss of family and friends, declining physical and mental health, etc. Some

people need help from health and social services for any or all of the following reasons:

- they gather a collection of problems which, together, are intolerable;
- they suffer particularly severe difficulties;
- they experience a sudden problem such as bereavement or crisis illness, which disturbs their normal methods of coping.

5 People in good health and with an adequate income are much less likely to find old age a time of problems.

WHERE TO LEARN MORE

There is a vast and growing gerontological literature. Much of it is American and can be heavy going, as well as being of doubtful relevance to what happens in Britain.

A good place to start is with what the carers have to say. Read the account referred to earlier by Slack and Mulville (1987) and those collected together by Briggs and Oliver (1985) of the experiences of carers. Put together with the descriptions by elderly people referred to in the previous chapter (see pp. 9–11), these give a good basic insight. They are also interesting to read!

Recent introductions to gerontology and to social policy and ageing are:

Bromley, D. B. (1988) *Human Ageing: An Introduction to Gerontology*, Harmondsworth: Penguin Books. This is the third edition of a wide-ranging and widely used textbook which is mainly about the psychology of ageing but paints a very broad backcloth.
Phillipson, C. and Walker, A. (1986) *Ageing and Social Policy: A Critical Assessment*, Aldershot: Gower. A collection of papers about policy and practice topics. It takes a critical and radical view and gives a stimulating introduction.

Chapter Three

WHAT ARE HOMES FOR?

So far the emphasis has been on ageing and the needs and experiences of elderly people. This is essential background to understanding how to help them and especially to understanding what residential Homes are intended to do for them and others.

It has been said that we must first decide what residential Homes are for and then arrange to achieve that as well as we can.

This seems a good place to start a more detailed look at Homes for elderly people: we need to be clear about our aims, objectives and goals. Unless we know where we are going we will not even know which direction to go in, let alone recognize it when we get there! In this chapter there is an introductory discussion of the purposes of Homes and other specialist accommodation and the ways they have developed.

EXPLAINING AND DESCRIBING HOMES

We can first *explain* Homes in the sense of exploring the purposes they are intended to serve for different people and groups: in part, this can be done through looking at the historical development of residential institutions. We must also be able to *describe* Homes – what they do, whom they do it for and how we will actually recognize a 'home' or 'Home'. The next chapter will go on to look at what Homes look like: how they have been described and some of their main characteristics.

The explanations that people have given for the development of institutions have been broadly built around three basic ideas:

1 There has been a general agreement that institutions of a

wide variety of types and purposes – such as prisons, psychiatric hospitals, and Homes for children and elderly people – all have some fundamental elements which are common. In some ways, all institutions are similar.

2 Perhaps the most dominant theme in the explanations has been the argument that institutions are intended to control. The elements of this argument are complex and wide-ranging. They have their origins in views that the development of the workhouse was mainly to support capitalism's need for a system to discourage some from avoiding work and also to control and discipline those who had no work. The growth of 'asylums' was seen as having a similar purpose of controlling and limiting those people whose behaviour was disturbing, disruptive or different.

3 Control explanations have been interlaced with those which take a more humanitarian view. Justifications are often based on a sense of obligation or duty to provide care or to 'meet the needs' of vulnerable people. This is characterized by the persistent view that residential care should be a last resort for elderly people who should be enabled to remain in their own homes for as long as possible.

A mixture of purposes

Institutions, therefore, are concerned with such things as restraint, restriction, punishment and control, as well as with such things as treatment, care, rehabilitation and support. Some kinds of institutions are more obviously about control and others about care or rehabilitation. Most, however, have an uneasy mix of purposes: some more openly understood and expressed than others.

There is no easy way to account for the existence of residential Homes. A number of studies have attempted to do so in detail and at length (see, in particular, Jones and Fowles 1984; Parker 1988). For the present purposes it is enough to know that there is a variety of explanations and there are sometimes conflicting reasons for residential care: both its general role in society and its purpose for each individual elderly person. We often find that Homes are wrestling with the need to control as well as to enable, to restrict as well as to rehabilitate. The mixed feelings of staff, residents and their family and friends can be traced back to the more fundamental ambivalences in society as a whole about whether institutions are to limit or to help those who live in them.

This is even more complicated when extended to thinking about the variety of forms of sheltered accommodation in which elderly people now live and receive help and support.

WHERE DO HOMES 'FIT'?

It may help to think about the part that residential Homes play in the overall range of services.

Government policy towards elderly people was set out in a White Paper, *Growing Older*, in 1981. This put emphasis on the desirability of people remaining in their own homes for as long as possible. This is a consistent theme of policy statements.

Another central theme has been the need to create an overall 'shape' to services to make sure that the right people get help and that as many people as possible get the best out of the help available. This has often been called the 'balance' of care.

This idea of finding a balance or shape to services is important at both national and local levels. Creating the most appropriate balance-of-care services in local areas probably depends on:

- Good local *information*: those who plan and manage services need a good basis of information from which to plan. Those who want to use services need to know the choices open to them.
- A *systematic planning strategy*: there should be a clear set of goals and a plan for how to reach them. This is only likely to work if all the different agencies (Social Services, Housing, Health, Leisure, etc.) agree the goals and plans and work together.
- Effective *management*: clear goals for putting plans into operation. It is generally agreed that Social Services provisions must be based on sound assessments and should be built up to meet the individual needs of elderly people to enable them to choose from a range of options.

The challenge to managers and practitioners alike is to make sure that scarce resources are spread as helpfully as possible amongst a lot of people in need. This involves some difficult decisions about whether to give relatively few very dependent people a high level of service or to offer less extensive help to a larger number of people in the hope that this will prevent them from becoming more dependent.

Residential Homes have a part to play in this balancing of priorities. There are decisions to be made, for instance, about whether to provide permanent care for very dependent people without family or community supports or to offer short periods of care for those who normally live with families or who cope with a great deal of support from family or friends. If short-stay care is provided, then there is a need to think about what kind of care is most helpful and for whom – and in what kinds of Homes it is best provided.

There are also important issues about the balance of public- and independent-sector provisions. These have become much more important in recent years. How will this balance be decided? Can it be left to market forces or will some agency or group need to take a lead? Is this a role for Local Authorities or for some other body?

These are some of the basic problems of deciding where residential Homes 'fit' into the overall pattern of services. A brief review of some of the historical background that has led to our present diversity of accommodation and care will help to set the issues in context.

HISTORICAL ASPECTS

The very early history of provision for elderly people in this country is one of voluntary care and especially care provided by the church. Monastic infirmary almshouses were the main provision for elderly people until the Reformation. Following the Dissolution of the Monasteries, those sick, elderly and needy people who could have relied on the church became homeless and destitute. In 1601 a Poor Law Act placed the responsibility for the care of the needy on the parishes and, for the next 300 years or so, care was provided in workhouses in which a mix of young, old, blind, mentally ill, sick and disabled people were cared for together.

From the end of the eighteenth century, the parishes increasingly adopted a system of supplementing low wages on a scale regulated by the price of bread. This eventually had the effect of reducing many of the ordinary working people to the position of paupers. The Poor Law Amendment Act of 1834 grouped parishes into Unions under the supervision of Boards of Guardians. This Act also made the workhouses, which were widely established by then, a general provision: outdoor relief (help outside the workhouse) could be given only to the sick, elderly people, widows and children; relief was available to the able-bodied only in the workhouse. The implication, therefore, was that an atmosphere of strict discipline would discourage the able-bodied poor from applying for help and would drive them to stay away from the workhouses. There were some charitably maintained almshouses, but most institutional care for older people was based on the Utilitarian attitude to the undeserving poor.

By the latter part of the nineteenth century as much as a third of the population had to resort to Poor Relief at some time in their lives. In 1908 the first old age pension was introduced and in 1925 this was extended by the principle of social insurance. Payment to elderly people then became, in theory, a return from contributions rather than a charitable payment from the state. In 1929 the Local Government Act transferred the powers of the Boards of Guardians to the County and Borough Councils, which were permitted to reclassify some of the institutions as hospitals. The widespread unemployment of the interwar years played a major part. The Unemployment Act of 1934 transferred responsibility for relief of the unemployed to central government and the financial reasons for deterrent policies in Poor Law institutions disappeared with this separation of responsibility for residential provision from that for financial relief.

1940s-50s

Changes and upheavals in traditional social relationships during the Second World War exposed a great deal of need and new attitudes led to the establishment of the National Health Service. Residential care was developed following the National Assistance Act in 1948.

In the immediate postwar years and the early 1950s, shortage of building materials and government restrictions on capital expenditure hindered the building of new establishments. Elderly people continued to be cared for in 'upgraded' workhouse institutions or in converted premises. Usually, the latter were large, older houses with steep stairs and no lifts, and often with big bedrooms sleeping five, six or more residents. In 1954 a review of Homes for elderly people was undertaken and this led to a recommendation that Homes for up to 60 residents should be built, especially where demand was heavy and sites few in the more populated areas (Ministry of Health 1955). At the same time other studies were showing up a shortage of places in residential accommodation and there were also practical difficulties of determining whether chronically sick older people should be cared for in hospital or residential accommodation. The Ministry took the view that long-term building should not begin until more was known about the effect of the development of geriatric care on overall need. The Phillips Committee (1954) emphasized the need for the development of domiciliary care and the importance of people in institutions retaining a community orientation. Three years later, a government circular (Ministry of Health 1957) approved these views and made an attempt to redefine the distinctions between hospital and residential care.

1960s

After the 1959 Mental Health Act, Local Authorities had power to provide residential accommodation for the mentally infirm and this, combined with a lifting of capital restrictions, encouraged an increase in building until Townsend's (1962) attack on the emphasis on residential provision in *The Last Refuge.*

Townsend's work was a milestone in the development of thinking about Homes. He was very critical of what was happening and referred especially to:

- Gross inequalities between different types of Homes.
- The shortcomings of Homes opened in the first 15 years after the war.
- The fact that the majority of people in Homes were not so handicapped or infirm that they could not live in homes of their own in ordinary accommodation with small amounts of help from domiciliary services from the community.
- The uneven quality of relationships between staff, family, friends and elderly people: Townsend stressed the importance of attitudes and the need to preserve and promote the elderly

person's power of self-determination through good health, adequate income, occupation, independent housing, etc.

Townsend concluded that Homes which existed at that time did not adequately meet the physical, psychological or social needs of elderly people. He advocated alternative services and living arrangements. In effect this meant developments in domiciliary social services, especially personal and domestic support in people's own homes and in special housing.

The question of who should provide continuous nursing care for those elderly people who needed it also still remained. The increasing emphasis in residential accommodation was on the needs of frail elderly people and this brought out additional issues about the need to employ people with nursing qualifications and night attendants.

Another important milestone which, although focused on hospital care, had a significant effect on thinking about institutions was Robb's book *Sans Everything* (1967). This was an attack on the conditions of hospital care of elderly people in psychiatric and geriatric hospitals. Barbara Robb expressed it simply and tellingly: 'We have to ask ourselves: are we really content to have our ailing grandparents living in prison-like circumstances? And do we want to face the prospect of ending up in this way ourselves?' (p. 8).

By the mid-1960s the major emphasis of policy statements was being placed on care in the community through improved and extended domiciliary health and welfare services. In 1968 a further government social survey (Harris 1968) indicated that many older people are admitted to care because of unsuitable alternative accommodation. A Ministry memorandum to Local Authorities and hospitals set out broad categories of people for whom they might normally expect to have to provide accommodation. It also suggested that the right way to deal with those who were wrongly placed was to accept the status quo for those already in Homes but to try to avoid wrong placement, in the future, by joint planning.

By the end of the 1960s, therefore, most of the main themes that have dominated subsequent institutional provision for elderly people were in place. These included:

- The importance attached to community care or 'care in the community' as a cornerstone of policy.

- The assumption that domiciliary services and residential accommodation are a part of a continuum of provision.
- The role of residential Homes in providing increasingly for the most frail elderly people.
- The difficulties of the boundaries between nursing care and other kinds of personal support. Linked with this, the problems arising from the overlaps and administrative boundaries between health and social services – especially between long-stay hospitals and Homes. The importance attached, therefore, to joint planning of services.

1970s

The late 1960s and early 1970s saw a spurt of growth in numbers of Local Authority Homes. These tended to be rather smaller than those built in the previous ten years: generally, they were for around 40 residents and built with a greater variety of design. By the mid-1970s, however, building began to come to a halt with the imposition of restrictions on capital developments in the public sector.

In 1977 a DHSS memorandum was published which gave guidance on health care arrangements in Local Authority Homes for elderly people. It set out what was to be the most substantial guidance for the following decade – not only about health and personal care boundaries, but also more generally about the purpose and function of residential Homes in the public sector:

Residential Homes are primarily a means of providing a greater degree of support for those elderly people no longer able to cope with the practicalities of living in their own homes even with the help of the domiciliary services. The care provided is limited to what might be provided by a competent and caring relative able to respond to emotional as well as physical needs. It includes, for instance, help with washing, bathing and dressing; assistance with toilet needs; the administration of medicines and, when a resident falls sick, the kind of attention someone would receive in his own home from a caring relative under guidance of the general practitioner or nurse member of the primary health care team. However, the staff of a Home are not expected to provide the professional kind of health care that is properly the function of the primary health care services. Nor should residential homes be used as nursing homes or extensions of hospitals.

(DHSS/Welsh Office 1977)

This was the basis of the public – Local Authority – provision of residential care by the late 1970s. The development of institutional care had moved through a series of stages. Sometimes it was influenced by a spirit of public generosity and will to provide a better life for 'the old and needy'. Sometimes it was more directed by the need to provide as cheaply as possible from scarce resources. Usually it was based on an uneasy compromise of these two motivations.

From an entirely charitable provision there was a move through a philosophy of strict workhouse provision, designed to discourage rather than to care, to the developments of the latter half of the twentieth century. Immediately after the National Assistance Act provision was in adapted accommodation. Through the 1950s and early 1960s larger purpose-built Homes were developed, to be followed by a period of quite extensive building of rather smaller Homes.

By the mid-1970s the great majority of accommodation was owned and run by the Local Authorities who were also diversifying in the provision of an increasing range of community support services: meals-on-wheels, luncheon clubs, day centres, home helps, etc.

Since that time, a number of significant developments have taken place which need to be explored in more detail if we are to have a full understanding of the present scene and 'who does what and why'. In particular, we need to look at:

- the rapid extension of private-sector provision;
- the development of a range of alternative, more flexible and innovative types of provision (from sheltered and very sheltered housing to resource and community support units);
- the changing perception of residential Homes within the range of choices for elderly people;

- the increasing awareness of the needs of carers: those people who provide help and support to elderly friends and relatives in the community.

RECENT DEVELOPMENTS: THE INDEPENDENT SECTOR

In the ten years from 1975 to 1986 there was only a very small rise in the numbers of Local Authority Homes (from 2,459 to 2,668). There was also little change in the number of Homes run by voluntary bodies. In the same period, however, the numbers of privately owned Homes rose very substantially. In 1975 there were 1,770 private Homes; this increased to 6,099 in 1986, by which time private homes represented more than three-fifths of the total number of all Homes. The increase in their numbers was particularly marked after 1980.

Several reasons have been given for this growth. Underlying all the development is the growth of the number of older people. The population of people over retirement age grew, nationally, from 5.5 million in 1951 to almost 8.5 million in 1981. These figures hide within them a particularly significant growth in recent years in the numbers of people over 75 and especially over 85: these are the groups now most likely to be entering residential care.

The financial limitations on Local Authorities described above have prevented all but a few from building any new Homes themselves since the mid-1970s.

Particularly significant in the private-sector development was the change in DHSS benefit rules in 1983 which enabled the government to pay the charges for people in private Homes up to a set local (later national) limit. Throughout Great Britain, the numbers of people claiming Supplementary Benefit Board and Lodging Allowance in private and voluntary Homes – the majority caring for elderly people – rose from 7,000 in 1979 to 90,000 in 1986 (Gibbs and Bradshaw 1987a).

This startling growth in the size of the independent sector presented difficulties for the Local Authority Social Services Departments who had the duty of registering private and voluntary Homes, and for the District Health Authorities who registered Nursing Homes. In 1984 the Registered Homes Act brought together the legislation for Nursing Homes and what were now called Residential Care Homes. It introduced more stringent requirements for registration and inspection and for the running of Homes.

Associated with the Act were new regulations and a code of practice – *Home Life* – for Residential Care Homes (Centre for Policy on Ageing 1984). A code was also produced by the National Association of Health Authorities for the District Health Authorities. *Home Life* was written by a working party convened by the Centre for Policy on Ageing at the request of the DHSS. It was to form the basis of the Local Authorities' approach to registration and inspection, although it was advisory rather than obligatory. It deliberately avoided making prescriptions on the grounds that what might be seen as appropriate care in one Home might not be right for another. Nevertheless, it did set out basic principles of care and then went on to describe good practice in social care, physical features of the Home, staffing matters, and the role of the registration authority. It also set out some elements which were relevant to particular groups of people living in homes.

Referring to elderly people, *Home Life* makes the important and fundamental point:

> Within one home, age may vary by as much as 30 years, though most people will be over 75. Personalities, interests, tastes, accustomed life-style and levels of physical and mental health will be extremely diverse . . . residential homes catering for older people should put maximum emphasis on enabling residents to manage their own lives to the greatest attainable extent and so make it possible for them to maintain their dignity, their independence, and their previous lifestyle.

Residential Care Homes in the independent sector (both private and voluntary) are registered and inspected by the Social Services Department. Nursing Homes are registered and inspected by the District Health Authority. It is possible for a Home to register dually, to provide both residential care and nursing facilities; however, only relatively few Homes have done so since it became possible in 1984. The main purpose of introducing dual registration was to enable people to be cared for in the same Home when they become sick.

The much extended role of the registering authorities presented them with a more difficult and challenging task. There is much yet to be learned about the purposes and potential of this regulating system. It offers the potential to provide both controls and developmental support to Homes.

RECENT DEVELOPMENTS: THE SPECTRUM OF PROVISION

One of the difficulties of discussing services for elderly people is that 'the elderly' cannot possibly be considered as a single group with a distinct set of needs. Ten million people cannot have identical needs: what is necessary is a range and variety of provisions to meet the many and varied requirements of those older people who do need help in their daily lives. To understand the purpose and potential of residential care, it has to be set in the context of the wider service provisions.

The range of proper provision will include income support, special housing, promotion and maintenance of good health, support for family and friends caring for older people, as well as the range of personal Social Services provision – residential care, home helps, meals services, day care, etc.

The Audit Commission for Local Authorities in England and Wales carries out 'value for money' exercises on Local Authorities: its task is to promote 'efficiency, effectiveness and economy' in services. In 1985 it produced a report on *Managing Social Services for the Elderly More Effectively*. The report was a substantial study of the ways in which the services provided by Social Services Departments for elderly people interrelate with each other to meet the needs of the most appropriate people (those in greatest need and/or who are most likely to benefit) in the most efficient and effective ways.

The report points out that any move to substantially increase residential care facilities would create an enormous resource problem. Some of the pressures for more residential provision are eased, however, because of the belief of many people engaged in helping elderly people that the well-being of older people is best served by supporting them in the community for as long as possible. If unnecessary or premature admission to residential care can be avoided without exposing people to unnecessary risk, the Audit Commission suggests, the result will be greater value for money for the elderly person as well as for the ratepayers.

The report goes on to identify some particular weaknesses in the way services are run. These will be explored in more detail later and are listed only briefly here to illustrate some of the issues:

- some people are 'inappropriately placed' in residential care;
- community services are not always directed to those who need them most;
- there is sometimes inadequate co-ordination of health, housing and social services;
- there is inadequate management of community services (unclear objectives, inexplicit policies and guidelines, no systems for monitoring services).

A major issue for the development of the range of services for elderly people, then, is how to make the best use of existing services to help as many people as possible in the most useful and effective way we can. There is a wide and growing body of research on social services provisions and some of the findings will be introduced in later chapters. Some of the most important things for providing an effective range of services seem to be the need for good assessment; joint planning and collaboration between health and social services; the role of the home help service as the core provision in the community; and the role of residential Homes in providing for a core group of very elderly, highly dependent people.

In 1988 a report of a study by Sir Roy Griffiths for the Secretary of State for Social Services (Griffiths 1988) looked at how public funds were being used to support community care policies. Although about services in the community generally, the report made some important recommendations affecting services for elderly people.

The report drew attention to the difference between the social security system which is based on entitlement to benefit and is open-ended, and the social services approach which assesses people's needs and then decides what they will receive on the basis of agreed priorities and available budgeted provisions. The two approaches were described as diammetrically opposed: a particularly important point for later discussion in this book about full assessment for admission to residential care which had been an expectation for Local Authority Homes but not for private Homes.

The Griffiths Report did, however, point out that the

'unintended consequence' of social security support for private residential care had been to provide accommodation for large numbers of people, many of whom would probably have needed it.

The report placed some stress on a theme that has become more and more important in thinking about provision for elderly people: the need for packages of care, developed around individuals to meet their unique needs with the best effect in local circumstances:

> At local level the role of social services authorities should be reorientated towards ensuring that the needs of individuals within specified groups are identified, packages of care are devised and services coordinated; and where appropriate a specific care manager is appointed... As to residential accommodation, social services authorities should be responsible for assessing whether a move to such accommodation was in the best interests of the individual and what the local authority would be prepared to pay for.

The reports of the Audit Commission and of Sir Roy Griffiths brought out the main current issues in the range of provision for older people in the community. These include:

- the balance between the needs of a core group of heavily dependent, very elderly people and a larger group of less dependent people with varying needs;
- the need for co-ordination of health and community services, including housing;
- the need for good assessment to ensure that the right services reach the people who are most likely to benefit;
- the need for clear objectives, policies and guidelines and for regular monitoring to make sure that services are doing what they are intended to do for the people for whom they are designed.

These issues should be seen in the context of broad government policies which were set out in a White Paper in 1981 (DHSS 1981). This said that:

> The Government's overall priority is to reduce and contain inflation. No policy could be more helpful to elderly people. ... Money may be limited but there is no lack of human

resources. Nor is there any lack of good will. An immense contribution is already being made to the support and care of elderly people by families, friends and neighbours and by a wide range of private, voluntary and religious organisations. We want to encourage these activities so as to develop the broadest possible base of service.

Supporting elderly people, in other words, is also very much about supporting those people who provide them with day-to-day care in their own homes.

A further White Paper published in 1989 (Department of Health 1989) broadly accepted the majority of the Griffiths proposals and set a new agenda for the development of community care for the following decade. This included new arrangements for paying for the care of residents in independent homes by the Local Authorities and for ensuring that elderly people have the opportunity of full assessment of their needs (including multidisciplinary assessment where necessary) so that residential care might become 'a positive choice'. The White Paper set out radical new expectations of the organization of services which will take some years to evolve.

RECENT DEVELOPMENTS: RESIDENTIAL CARE, ACCOMMODATION AND THE FUTURE

This background sets the scene for understanding the kinds of residential homes we have now and are likely to have in the future. The Local Authorities have a stock of Homes built mainly during the 20 years up to 1975, with some remaining older, adapted Homes. These are all presenting a growing problem of maintenance of the buildings themselves. The private sector has grown enormously in recent years and the relationship between this expanded resource and the Local Authorities who regulate and inspect it has yet to be fully developed.

In addition, there is a wide variety of sheltered housing, much of which provides care or support of a more or less limited kind on the premises. Sheltered housing expanded rapidly during the 1960s and 1970s alongside the growth of residential care. It was a new form of provision whose main contribution was that it enabled people to live in separate housing units, retaining privacy and control over their lives whilst having access to community care supports and, often, an emergency call system to a nearby warden which could give at least a feeling of security. It also offered scope for flexibility and experiment with building design.

The majority of the initial sheltered housing developments were built by the Local Authorities. More recently, housing associations and private-sector developments have begun to lead provision. About one-fifth of sheltered housing units are now provided by housing associations. Private units have become increasingly significant: some 20,000 were built by the end of 1986 (although these tend to be in the South of the country).

People who wish to remain in their own homes are now more likely to be able to get help to do so. Improvements in technology have enabled alarm and call systems to be installed in private housing. Building societies have begun to advance loans in which some or all of the interest is added to capital to be repaid only on death or sale of the house: the cost does not fall on the elderly person in her lifetime.

The range of housing options is therefore extending. The role of residential care in this changing scene has inevitably had to be carefully considered. At the end of 1985 an independent review of residential care was commissioned by the Secretary of State for Health and Social Services. A committee based at the National Institute for Social Work was set up and reported in 1988 (Wagner Report 1988)

The Wagner Report ranges widely across issues of good practice in all types of Homes. Some of these issues will be introduced later in this book. The report sets out important basic principles and, in particular, suggests that

> People who move into establishments should do so by positive choice. A distinction should be made between need for accommodation and need for services. No-one should be required to change their permanent accommodation in order to receive services which could be made available to them in their own homes.

The report makes particular mention of the needs of elderly people with mental infirmities. This is a very significant group, representing an increasingly high proportion of residents.

The Wagner Report served two important functions. First, it

summarized good practice assumptions and brought together ideas and knowledge about residential Homes from work with all client groups. Second, it promoted a positive view of residential care and its potential to help people when properly used within a range of other community resources and services.

It also helps to draw attention to the range of developments in residential provisions for elderly people: Homes offering various forms of group living arrangements, the growth of small Homes in the private sector, innovative developments in using Homes as resource centres to offer day care, meals, a base for community groups and workers, etc. It is clearly no longer appropriate to think of residential Homes as one form of care. There is a range and variety which needs to be approached with flexibility and creativity.

There is, however, a substantial central core of residential provision in which elderly people receive a good deal of personal care throughout the day and night and in which they live with a large group of others in a relatively public, shared form of accommodation.

WHAT ARE HOMES FOR: KEY POINTS

This chapter has described the background to the broad and challenging scene in which Homes now exist. In that sense, it has tried to *explain* why we have the Homes we now have. Some key points should be stressed once again:

- Homes are intended to help people. They help older people by providing warmth, food, protection, etc. They also help others by taking the burden of care from family and friends and by containing the difficult behaviour of some mentally infirm people. They therefore have mixed and sometimes confused purposes and people often have a similarly mixed and confused attitude to them.
- Homes need to be seen in relation to all the other services that are available for elderly people. Their function is, in part, defined by their place in the wider spectrum of care services.
- There are lots of different sorts of Homes and care: different people need and want different things and a variety of choices is necessary and desirable.

WHERE TO LEARN MORE

There is still a good deal to be learned from Peter Townsend's (1962) work, described earlier. *The Last Refuge* still has a lot to teach us about Homes, their purposes and limitations.

The best summary of current good practice in residential Homes as a whole is the Wagner Report (1968). The second volume to the report includes a review of the historical background to residential care in general (by R. Parker) and a review of research on Homes for elderly people (by I. Sinclair). Both are invaluable summaries.

A much more technical and thorough discussion of the growth of social services for elderly people in Britain is available to anyone with the time and enthusiasm in:

Means, R. and Smith, R. (1985) *The Development of Welfare Services for Elderly People*, London: Croom Helm.

Chapter Four

WHAT DO HOMES DO?

The previous chapter sought to explain Homes by describing how they have developed and how they fit into the wider pattern of service provision.

Another way of beginning to establish what Homes are for is to look at what they actually *do*. Whatever the larger claims of policy and statements of philosophy, who actually goes into a Home and lives and dies there will really depend on the day-to-day purposes and wishes of the people who live and work there.

WHO GOES IN? A NOTE ON OPTIMISM AND REALISM

When the Association of Directors of Social Services presented their evidence to the Wagner Committee they said that the emphasis is now on residential care:

1 For those people for whom residential care is the only feasible way of providing the care and attention that they need.
2 For those individuals who choose residential care as an alternative living situation to any other proposed solution to their particular problems, having fully understood and considered alternatives.
3 Where individuals need a specifically tailored programme with specific aims which can only be provided on a residential basis and which is time limited, e.g. treatment, rehabilitation, assessment.
4 Where, in order to maintain an individual in their own home a period of respite is required for their carers.
5 Where an individual is ejected at a time of crisis from their

normal living situation and where a residential 'crash pad' is needed to permit alternative care plans to be developed.

(ADSS 1986)

In these terms, residential Homes funded by Local Authorities are to provide for people for whom there is no real option, for some people in emergency, and on a short-term basis for respite. They may also provide assessment and rehabilitation and may be where some people choose to be.

It would be nice to think that Homes for elderly people offer detailed assessment and rehabilitation and can make a contribution to community care plans. Certainly, large numbers of people now stay in Homes for planned short-stay periods for a variety of purposes, including assessment, rehabilitation and respite. The great majority of admissions to Local Authority Homes are now for short stays: probably in the order of three short-stay admissions to every long stay. It might once have been argued that few people entering the institutional system would ever leave it except through death. The picture is no longer so clear cut, particularly as around half of all places are in private or voluntary Homes which have a greater variety of patterns of care and residents.

However, it should be remembered that people entering residential care are now more likely than ever before to be very old and very frail. A high proportion have some degree of mental frailty. It is right that we should look with optimism for flexible ways of promoting opportunities for them to grow and develop when they are in Homes. We should not be blind to the real difficulties and limitations.

WHAT IS A HOME? DOMESTICITY AND INSTITUTIONALIZATION

In a sense, nobody needs residential care. What people need is food, warmth, security, companionship and the opportunity to do what they find fulfilling. People tend to think of 'home' as the place where they belong and where they can expect to get these physical and emotional needs met. The idea of home is therefore not just about environment and emotional needs. It is also about the way people feel about a particular place and what it means to them.

Mary Stott quotes a conversation with a little girl, a 'displaced person', in a refugee camp: '"We shall be able to find a home for you and your family soon". "Oh", said the child, "we've got a home. All we need is a house to put it in"' (Stott 1981: 11). This is a very helpful illustration of a fundamental difference between feeling at home in the sense of feeling at ease and 'belonging' and the place in which the home is located.

It has been argued (Willcocks *et al.* 1987) that in the past the basic mistake was trying to provide a domestic environment in an institutional building. It is not possible to make a large institution for 40 or 50 residents 'the same as' a family home. In Homes large groups of people come together as strangers to share long periods of the day in public lounges and dining rooms, only retiring to private rooms to sleep. This is far from the familiar family life-style which most of them will previously have enjoyed (at some time, even if not immediately before going into the Home).

The ideas of home and domesticity contrast sharply with the ways in which institutions actually work. Residential institutions, whether hospitals, prisons or residential Homes, have an internal life of their own. Each has an organized social system which is maintained by all those who live and work in it: everyone quickly learns the spoken and unspoken expectations and rules of daily living and acts within them – or suffers the consequences.

One of the most useful and widely used contributions to thinking about institutions remains that of Goffman (1961). In *Asylums* he suggests that institutions have an all-encompassing – or, in Goffman's term, 'total' – character which is symbolized by barriers to interaction with the society outside the institution. Often, he suggests, these barriers are physically built into the structure of the institution in the form of locked doors or high walls. They may also be implicit in other restrictions such as limit-ations on coming and going and outside contacts. He lists the total institutions in our society in five rough groupings. First, there are those established to care for people who are both incapable and felt to be harmless (e.g. Homes for the old, the blind, etc.). Second, there are institutions caring for incapable people who may present a threat to others (e.g. psychiatric hospitals). Third, there are those which contain people who present intentional dangers (e.g. prisons). Other institutions are established to pursue working tasks more effectively and, finally, some are designed as retreats from the world.

Goffman's concept of the 'total institution' has several central features. All aspects of life – sleeping, eating, working and playing – are carried out in the same place under the same control; all daily living activities have to happen in the company of others who tend to be treated alike; all phases of the day's activities are tightly scheduled; and all activities are brought together in a single plan to fulfil the official aims of the institution.

Jones and Fowles (1984) point out that the only first-hand evidence available to Goffman was from one atypical mental hospital. His grounds for making generalized statements were based on what they regard as a selective use of a wide range of sources. Reviewing a selected group of key research reports on institutions with very different purposes they conclude that there is a basic theme to all the work. They suggest the theme has five main aspects. Namely, institutional care is characterized by:

- loss of liberty;
- social stigma;
- loss of autonomy;
- depersonalization;
- low material standards.

They argue that the idea of a 'total institution' is misleading because no institution is totally cut off from the rest of the world. Each must therefore be subject to some influences and be shaped by the outside world to a degree. In Goffman's terms, however, it may be experienced as 'total' by the person living there if he is totally cut off from outside contact and subject to the institution's pervading restrictions and controls. As Jones and Fowles (1984: 203) graphically put it:

the basic recognition 'I cannot get out, I am like these people I see around me, I cannot make my own decisions' is not really modified by spring mattresses and cheerful curtains; but when bleakness, deprivation and squalor are added to helplessness, any institution becomes a punishment block.

One other perspective will be helpful. Russell Barton described the effects of living in an institution as if they could be thought of as an illness which he called 'institutional neurosis'. The patient or resident becomes highly dependent. Apathy and withdrawal result from an erosion of personality. Typically the posture of the elderly person in an institution was said to show common effects: slumped in a chair, head bowed and with little facial expression, taking no interest in nearby events. These behaviours are associated with the negative elements of an enclosed life: ritualized behaviour of staff and residents, rigidity of rules, lack of privacy, lack of stimulation and enforced idleness, loss of personal friends, possessions and significant day-to-day experiences, and loss of hope and opportunity. They may often be aggravated by the effects of medication.

Homes for elderly people can vary considerably in the extent to which they show these traits of institutions in extreme forms. Many approximate in some ways to domestic characteristics and can meet the needs of individual residents if the environmental and group pressures and processes are properly understood and managed.

Barton described some typical ways of behaving by using medical terminology. Whether or not they are described in illness terms is not important. The tendency to behave in fixed, habitual ways and to become withdrawn and apathetic are common features of institutional life. The five factors stressed by Jones and Fowles are central to a view of how to strive to offset some of the worst effects on individuals. For example:

Institutional features	*Indications for potential action*
Loss of liberty	Ensure mobility, opportunities for free movement inside and outside the Home and access to community facilities.
Social stigma	Encourage feelings of self-worth by providing valued activities and social interactions with others.
Loss of autonomy	Ensure respect for individual rights: privacy, choice, self-control, etc.
Depersonalization	Treat people as individuals (e.g. learn how they wish to be addressed; individual care plans; freedom of choice and opportunity).
Low material standards	Good design; making creative use of what is available; decorating to resident's choice.

70

REGIME AND LIFE-STYLES

Another way of looking at this is to think about how to describe what goes on within Homes on a daily basis. This has sometimes been called the 'regime' of the Home

It is when we begin to consider the regimes of Homes that the enormous variety of life-styles to be found becomes clear. The existence of this variety makes it obvious that the search for the 'common' elements in institutions described above is sterile without an appreciation of the ways in which unique environments affect individuals differently. In other words, it may be helpful to have a basic understanding of what happens generally in institutions but each Home must be understood in terms of its distinct and different impact on each resident.

There are basically six factors which contribute to making up the life-style of the Home:

1 The individuals who live there: with their individual and shared life experiences, their separate needs, personalities and wishes.
2 The staff who work there: each also bringing their own experiences and expectations.
3 The rules, routines and habits of daily life in the Home: the way in which the social and personal interactions are organized.
4 The physical environment, especially the building, its furnishings and decoration: offering potentials and limitations to the ways people interact and behave in their daily life experience.
5 The relationships between people who live there and those who work there: their attitudes and behaviour towards each other.
6 The relationships between the people who live and work there with the world outside the Home: interaction with the community, use of the normal facilities of the world beyond the Home.

Think, for a moment, about which if any of these factors constitute the sense of 'home'. The character and atmosphere of daily experience will probably be made up of the interaction of all of them. In order to understand what Homes do, it is necessary to think about each of these six dimensions.

Overall, however, most of us have an idea of what 'a good Home' should be just as we have an idea of a good hotel, a good shop, etc. Some writers have described Homes by relating them to other sorts of establishments. Some of these 'models' may help to clarify what a Home should be doing. *A Home may be said to be:*

(1) Like a hotel. A hotel is a place where you can rent a private room for living, sleeping and eating, although usually some important activities of life, such as relaxing, socializing and eating, are carried out in public rooms. In return for payment, staff carry out various tasks – cleaning, laundry, creating and serving meals, etc. In many ways this resembles residential care: accommodation and services are also provided for a charge. Yet it is quite common to hear staff say in a critical way of a resident, 'She treats this place like a hotel.' This needs to be thought through carefully when planning what kind of place a Home should be. A resident viewed as a customer – a buyer of services – is likely to be seen as more powerful than when seen in terms of the more common view of residents as passive recipients. Such a view may be of considerable advantage to residents.

(2) Like a warehouse. Homes have sometimes been seen as warehouses in the sense that they are places where elderly people are 'stored' until death. This is a particularly negative and depersonalizing way of looking at things. Sadly, it is not difficult to find Homes in which residents receive little stimulation or opportunity. Physical care may often be good but social stimulation limited: the result is apathy, disinterest and 'storage'.

(3) Like a hospital. Hospitals are primarily to provide medical treatment for sick people. In a strict sense residential Homes do not do this. Nursing Homes do provide nursing and medical care for people who are ill and have a lot of features in common with residential Homes. The distinction between nursing and personal care is a complicated but important one and will be discussed in more detail later. Many people in Homes are physically frail and do need some medical help but Homes are not hospitals. There is a sense in which they are similar in that both offer rehabilitation: an encouragement to people to develop or relearn skills to enable them to lead a more active life.

(4) Like a psychogeriatric ward. A high proportion of elderly

people in many Homes have some degree of mental disorder, commonly dementia. Shifts in hospital practices leading to higher turnover of patients, less in-patient and more out-patient and day-care provision have had an impact on residential Homes. Many are, therefore, providing for people who need help with psychiatric needs.

These are just some of the possible models which offer perspectives on regimes. Aspects of each may feature to a degree in most Homes. The important issues are that those running the Homes should have thought through the purposes of the Home, the implications of the life-style they are creating, the influences on it and its impact on residents. The creation of a life-style should be purposeful.

MEASURING REGIMES

Perhaps the most substantial work on regimes in Britain has been that of Booth (1985). Although writing with a research orientation his comments on how to assess, measure or evaluate the character of a Home are helpful in beginning to understand how to affect and use life-styles to help people. He makes four basic points about the perspectives that might be taken in the process of measuring or evaluating what is going on in a Home:

1 Deciding whether it is the individual dimensions (physical, social or interpersonal) of the environment which are the most significant or whether the institution has some overall character – an integrated whole – which can be recognized and evaluated.
2 Deciding whose perspective to adopt: that of the staff, the residents, an observer or some combination. Who has the right to decide whether it is a good home?
3 Deciding whether to focus on how people feel about their situation or on a set of objective features.
4 Selecting between people's attitudes, their patterns of behaviour, the policies of the organization and the actual caring practices as the way of distinguishing differences between Homes.

Booth developed an Institutional Regimes Questionnaire. This is made up of 31 multiple-choice questions about different aspects of the management and organization of everyday life in a Home. These provide a basis for comparing Homes on four main areas of daily life through scales measuring:

1 Personal choice: based on variables such as bedtimes, getting up, breakfast-times, menu choice and planning, access to grounds, furniture, decoration, refreshments, alcohol, personal allowances and meetings.
2 Privacy: based on variables such as access to grounds and beyond, locking bedrooms, personal valuables and access to bedrooms.
3 Segregation: based on access beyond the grounds, locking front door, visitors, overnight accommodation, telephone, away visits, social activities, entertainment, outings, holidays.
4 Participation: based on menu-planning, domestic tasks, home entertainment and meetings.

These scales begin to introduce some of the central issues which are essential to being able to answer questions such as:

- Are the routines of the Home flexible or structured?
- Is the regime responsive or unresponsive to individual needs and wishes?
- Is the environment open or closed to interaction and outside influences?
- Is the regime autocratic or democratic in its attention to residents' involvement and decision-making?

HOW DO REGIMES AFFECT PEOPLE: WHAT IS IMPORTANT?

If we are to be able to go on to judge the right way of running Homes it will be helpful to begin to introduce some more detailed distinctions about the quality of the service provided.

The definition and measurement of quality of life in Homes has been developed around several dimensions: especially happiness (how people feel about their lives and whether they express satisfaction) but with a more recent recognition that the well-being of individuals has to be looked at from several directions to appreciate the full picture. Physical, psychological and social aspects must be measured and understood to build up the full picture.

There are two main things to be taken into account in order to understand the assessment of quality of Homes. First, there are all the resources of the Home (its design, staffing levels, food, warmth, etc.) and the ways in which staff behave, their attitudes and skills. These together make up what we generally call 'care' provision. Second, there is the impact of that care on the residents and the way in which they experience the quality of their lives in the Home.

When thinking about the quality of residential Homes, therefore, it will be helpful to distinguish between the *quality of care* and the *quality of life*. Quality of care will be used here to refer to the quality of the resources and activities managed in the process of providing residential care. Quality of life will be used to refer to the benefits experienced by consumers as a result of these care inputs. It is the relationship between the two – what we know about the effects of particular types of care on the quality of life for residents – that is fundamental to good residential work practice.

What we know about the effects of residential life on people can, therefore, be discussed in these two broad dimensions of quality of care and quality of life. The preceding discussion of institutionalization and the nature of regimes has identified the range of general deficiencies that commonly occur in quality of care. In a summary of research in this area, a National Institute for Social Work report (NISW 1988) concluded that the most significant deficiencies cluster around three main themes:

- Lack of choice: this applies in different ways at almost every point in the application for residential care and then is equally apparent in life after entering a Home.
- Lack of security(legal and psychological): this, the report argues, has a substantial effect on a resident's sense of well-being before and after entering a Home.
- Absence of any real sense of control over their own lives is experienced by elderly people: although true for many elderly people in their own homes this is much more the case in residential Homes.

The NISW report stresses a further factor: the relative if not absolute lack of power of elderly people to influence decisions taken about entry to care and about many aspects of life in Homes.

In fact, the evidence about whether regimes affect residents' levels of satisfaction, or well-being, or health in any substantial way is very confusing. There is a considerable weight of support in professional literature and 'good practice' statements such as *Home Life* (Centre for Policy on Ageing 1984) and the Wagner Report (1988) for the view that the lack of choice, power, security and control over personal decision-making leads to increased dependency and other problems in functioning in residents. There is a dominant view, in other words, that what would be readily recognized as oppressive regimes tend to produce dependent residents.

The research evidence is far less conclusive. Booth (1985: 220), for instance, concluded from research in four English Local Authorities that

> Existing differences between regimes had no more than a marginal effect on the functioning of residents and differences in outcome were unrelated to the characteristics of the regimes. . . Regimes that allow residents less freedom are no more likely to increase their dependency than others.

In a review of research on the effectiveness of social care for elderly people, Goldberg and Connelly (1982: 213) summarized nine features of residential Homes which are held to make the quality of life better:

1 flexibility of management practices
2 individualization and autonomy for residents
3 opportunities for privacy
4 opportunities for social stimulation
5 communication and interaction with the world outside
6 social interaction between staff and residents . . .
7 maximum delegation of decision-making to care staff and to residents
8 good communication channels between staff
9 a minimum degree of specialization of roles and tasks among staff.

There is, however, little clear, *direct* relationship between these and residents' well-being. They clearly have a relationship to the things we value: independence, respect, dignity, etc. Indirectly they are likely to be related to the overall feeling of satisfaction, but there is not a lot of research evidence for this.

I. Sinclair (1988) reviewed much of the relevant research for the Wagner Committee. He concluded that quality of life, as perceived by the resident, can probably be best assessed according to the way in which it meets basic needs for physical and medical care, allows residents control over key aspects of their lives and counteracts loneliness and boredom.

It is difficult for researchers to get an accurate view of how residents feel for at least two reasons. First, elderly people usually express satisfaction with what they have got in a general sense (although often residents will say, 'You've got to like it, haven't you?'), perhaps because they have no real options to choose from or because, for residents especially, there is a fear of complaining and consequent reprisals. Second, different people want different things. Sinclair argues, however, that there are three main areas in which residents preferences are consistent:

1 They appreciate the comfort, physical security and freedom from worry that Homes can provide.
2 They want to control certain key aspects of their lives: e.g. to be private when they choose; to choose their own companions; to control their immediate physical environment, such as being able to open a window or vary room temperatures; and to have security and tenure.
3 They value company and interesting activities – if they are able to choose these for themselves.

There is, of course, a difference between knowing what they want and knowing whether these factors actually influence levels of satisfaction, well-being, dependency, survival or other objectively measurable features of quality of life. Booth's findings that regimes are not a major influence on dependency and functioning sound an important cautionary note but are not an argument for failing to respect the rights and meet the wishes of elderly individuals.

A CHECKLIST FOR GOOD CARE

What has begun to accumulate here is the makings of a checklist to state the assumptions and issues that influence good care practices. There is, however, no single way of running a 'good Home', since people want and need different things. No checklist could be adequate and might actually encourage inflexibility if it were interpreted as a description of the only 'right way' to run a Home. Sinclair's brief list of key 'wants' of residents is a good, simple starting-place for judging a Home and how to set about improving it.

Some basic questions should be:

1 Is the Home comfortable and are residents confident of their security and tenure in the Home?
2 Can the residents control key aspects of their daily life? For example:

- Can they open and shut windows in their rooms?
- Can they control heating and turn lights on and off?
- Do they have somewhere to lock up possessions?
- Can they lock their own room?
- Can (and do) they retain their own pension books and cash?
- Do they retain their own GP?
- Do they have a choice of food?

3 Is there a choice of activities and can residents choose whom to spend their time with?

PUTTING PRINCIPLES INTO PRACTICE: CREATING A HOME

There is a long tradition of thinking which recognizes the connections between a person's inner and outer worlds in institutions. Basically, this view proposes that an individual can be seen as having a set of 'competencies', perhaps most simply thought about as abilities to cope in the areas of health, physical functioning, intellectual ability and 'ego strength'.

At the same time the approach proposes that environments can be classified in terms of the direct demands they make on people. This has been called the 'environmental press'. An individual's experience of life in a given environment is said to be the result of the interaction between his competency and the environmental press: his ability to cope in relation to what is demanded of him by his surroundings (Lawton 1980).

The environment will be made up of

- the physical features;
- the social environment: rules, routines, regimes, etc.;
- the people and relationships.

These provide a useful framework for looking at how to put principles into practice.

PHYSICAL FEATURES: DESIGNING FOR CARE

The buildings in which residential care is located have a major effect on its quality, although it remains difficult to disentangle the effects on the quality of individual experiences.

There are probably two central questions:

- Do residents feel at ease or 'at home' in their surroundings?
- Can residents control their physical surroundings?

Homes come in a wide variety of shapes and sizes. Local Authority Homes changed gradually in design over a period of some 20 years from the late 1950s until the end of the 1970s, when the rate of building new Homes slowed down considerably. Probably around three-quarters have been purpose built, with some remaining converted, older properties, often with newer extensions. Over the years there has been a tendency to build Homes with fewer storeys but with more complicated ground plans (Peace 1986).

Private Homes tend to be smaller and some research has described the pressure to ensure that as much available space as possible is used for bedrooms (which can be rented) at the expense of public rooms – lounges and, especially, dining-rooms which cannot be used to produce extra income. Financial pressures also create other difficulties such as lack of handrails, which inhibits mobility in the Home (Judge *et al.* 1986).

With these issues and context in mind, some of the key features of designing a building to encourage and facilitate good care can be considered.

Size

Size is usually thought of in terms of the number of places for residents. Recent pressures have been towards smaller Homes on the principle that smallness more closely reproduces domesticity; there is also an assumption that good care principles can be more easily put into practice in smaller Homes. There are, however, economic pressures towards larger Homes. As Homes get bigger, the proportion of staff to residents tends to be lower and fosters a greater tendency to routines and less flexibility. Larger Homes may lead to more staff time being devoted to administration and management, to the detriment of resident care and direct contact.

On the other hand, larger Homes *could* offer a greater choice of people with whom to interact, although there is some evidence that this does not usually happen.

Location

The place in which a Home is sited is less important than that the people who live there have freely chosen to be there. A Home in a remote rural situation may be ideal for some but mean isolation and misery for others. Contact with the outside world and with community facilities is essential. If a Home is not close to shops, churches, pub, cinemas, etc., then goods and services may have to be brought in, making the Home more isolated and institutional.

Often it is the way they look rather than where they are sited that sets Homes apart from the locality and identifies them – and those who live there – as different. This contributes to the difference of life-style and can be offset in a number of ways: by design, by avoiding large identifying notices, etc. This can present dilemmas if private Homes feel the need to be visible to attract customers or voluntary Homes wish to encourage sympathy and fund-raising. It then becomes a matter of balancing competing priorities.

Public and private space

Some researchers have stressed the importance of the balance of what they call 'the public and the private space' (Peace *et al.* 1982). They have argued that,

> before entering a home people lead lives which are – to varying degrees – conducted partly in public and partly in

private, is it unreasonable to expect that the residential setting should permit the continuation of this pattern? Further-
more, should it be the individual resident who dictates the
balance of public and private, communal and individual life
he or she prefers?

Their survey of 100 Local Authority Homes found that residential
life is actually overwhelmingly public: residents tend to congregate
in dining-rooms and lounges. Private Homes often have a higher
proportion of private space but the pattern tends to be similar.

Peace and her colleagues were led to conclude that the focus of
life should be moved away from the public and communal towards
the personal and private. They felt there would need to be changes
in staff attitudes and in relationships with the community at large,
but particularly that the focal point of homes would need to
become the residential flatlet.

Lounges

The main public areas are usually the lounges. A good deal of
research has emphasized the importance of ensuring that there is
a choice of sitting area. Some, for instance, have stressed the need
to avoid centralized daytime accommodation which exposes
residents to continual staff surveillance and which encourages
queuing and group routines (Lipman and Slater 1977). Others
have reviewed the value of smaller 'group-living' designs which
would enable small numbers of perhaps six to eight to spend much
of their day together, visiting other groups by choice. This is
considered again later. What does seem of central importance is
that there should be a variety and choice of sitting area (preferably
with windows that can be seen through by people sitting down).

Corridors

Circulation areas can also be very important. They can be disorien-
tating if too similar to others in the establishment. They can be
tiring and discouraging if too long and without sitting or resting
places along the way. They can provide a safe area for confused
residents to walk freely.

Personal rooms

There is general agreement that most residents want single

bedrooms. Occasionally, married couples or others do choose to share and buildings should be flexible enough to allow this without imposing a shared room on strangers. A fundamental issue is the purpose of the room: is it a bedroom or does it have wider purposes? Can it be a bedsitting-room or flatlet from which the resident comes out for meals or to meet friends as she might from a flat or house? And can she control what happens in the room: can she open windows in safety, lock the door at any time, or say no to anyone wishing to clean if it is not convenient?

Accessibility

There should be free access in and out of Homes but also within the Home. Mealtimes can often create bottlenecks if narrow corridors lead to dining-rooms. In a wider sense residents need access to the outside world through views from windows and they should be able to see a variety of interesting things.

Decoration

The decoration should be clean and to the taste of those who live with it. It should be appropriate for the age group. Some thought should be given to the use of colours to help residents orientate themselves. If all the doors are faced in teak veneer then it is hardly surprising that residents go into the wrong rooms.

Floor coverings

The use of carpets is an important indication of attitudes to the environment. The problems of incontinence are sometimes said to make carpets undesirable. There are, of course, various makes of carpet which assist with this but the real problem is sometimes poor hygiene and care practices (wet clothing and sheets piled on carpets, poor continence management practices). A decision about the ways in which public and private areas are to be used may assist decisions about floor coverings. If a corridor is simply a short passageway from one private area to another then it may be regarded and carpeted differently than if it were an integral part of the 'home' and used for regular circulation and social interaction.

Furnishing

Many Homes have built-in furniture. Although this often makes more space available, it also restricts choice of arrangement and makes it more difficult to put an individual stamp on a room. It has been established that residents want to control their own environment. A basic way to achieve this is to provide them with an empty room and help them to furnish it as they wish.

Bathrooms and WCs

For many people, privacy of toilet facilities is the key to a more relaxed life. Problems can arise from centralized WCs, often in heavy demand during the day. Bathrooms should be near to bedrooms and should have ready access with special facilities for infirm or disabled residents.

Other design issues

These include the location of laundries where noise and smells do not intrude and soiled clothing is not trailed through the Home; the control of temperatures by residents to enable them to use all parts of the Home in comfort when they wish to do so; the need for an emergency call system; accessible location for night staff; and facilities to entertain visitors in private (that may quite simply mean providing comfortable chairs in personal rooms).

Physical features: some key questions

Access and opportunity

- Can residents use the kitchen area? What are the problems and potentials? If not, can they make a drink and snack elsewhere?
- Can residents get to all parts of the Home? Can wheelchair or walking-frame users use the WCs in private? Are light switches and TV sets, etc., accessible?
- Can residents use the laundry and other facilities of the Home to do things for themselves?

Privacy

- Can residents find a quiet place when they want? Can they lock the door? Can they lock valuables away safely? Who controls access to their rooms?

Safety

The balance between safety and protection and risk and choice is an important one which will be explored in detail later. From the design point of view two aspects are especially important:

- How is the balance of fire safety and resident needs and rights maintained? Are furnishings flameproof? Does this restrict resident choice? How do fire-doors affect residents' mobility?
- How safe is the general environment? Most accidents happen in bedrooms: what precautions are taken? Do these enhance or restrict residents' lives?

THE SOCIAL ENVIRONMENT: RULES AND ROUTINES

The daily experience of life in a Home for both residents and staff centres on a quite small number of routines. For residents these are mainly concerned with the basics of life and survival: sleeping, getting dressed, eating, keeping clean, going to the toilet. For staff, routines tend to be focused on a series of tasks, some linked to these basic needs of residents but others more generally related to keeping the establishment running: maintaining the building, ordering food and other necessary items, administering staff rotas, etc.

Typically, there are few staff to provide for the needs of a large group of residents. It is hardly surprising that when three Care Assistants and one Officer are available to meet the personal needs of 40 or more residents they tend to concentrate on essential tasks and do them in a habitual, routine way. This is seen to be necessary just to get through the day.

Chapter 2 discussed the importance of the exchanges that take place between people. Elderly residents need help and services. The more help they require the less likely it is that they will be able to control their own lives as they become subject to the routines of large group living. Staff tend to treat everyone in the same way for various reasons:

- the lack of time which creates pressures towards doing necessary tasks in minimal ways (as quickly as possible, with as little effort as possible);

- the concern to be fair: to make sure that no one is seen to get preferential treatment;
- anxieties about safety which lead, for example, to locking doors to prevent a handful of confused residents from wandering out but consequently restricting everyone, or to regular night-time checks on all residents whether they need them or not.

These are all real pressures. Meeting all the needs of a large group of individuals with limited time and resources is not possible. Decisions have to be made about priorities. Residential Homes can never be ideal for each individual when the needs of the one are in constant competition with the needs of the many.

Most Officers and staff of Homes would say, if asked, that there are few rules. They might list some basic safety rules: no smoking in bedrooms; fire-doors to be kept closed, etc. Hygiene rules may also be explicit: protective clothing; handling of food, etc. But they would probably identify few explicit, formal rules for the social life of the Home. Residents, on the other hand, can usually be very clear about a lot of commonly understood, informal rules: e.g. the TV in the main lounge is always left on ITV; no one can go out without informing a senior member of staff; relatives should not visit before 11 a.m.; pocket money is always given out on Friday morning; all medicines must be given to the head of Home.

Some kinds of routines are unavoidable: that is why Homes will always have some element of inflexibility and a depersonalizing effect on people who live there. This is a part of the deal elderly people have to make: they lose some personal control in return for security, physical help and other benefits. Nevertheless, many Homes have rules and expectations which are not necessary, in the sense that they are to meet the needs or concerns of staff rather than of residents. As a guiding principle, staff should try to ensure that their patterns of work are flexible enough to enable them to respond to individual residents' wishes.

The rest of this book explores ways of becoming, and remaining 'resident-centred'. For the present purposes, it will be helpful to note briefly some of the main areas around which routines develop and some of the questions to be addressed to avoid this.

Around the clock

For most residents, the day starts early. Usually, they are woken with a cup of tea, probably somewhere between 7 and 8 a.m. In private Homes the day may begin later and in a more relaxed fashion, perhaps with breakfast served in their rooms. In Local Authority Homes there is likely to be more of a rush. Some residents may be up and about before 7. Occasionally, this is through choice, sometimes the result of confusion about time, and sometimes because they went to bed too early the night before! There is a world of difference between waking everyone on a tea-round and providing a cup of tea to anyone who is awake or who has asked to be woken. Why should everyone get up at the same time? This can actually create pressures on staff, who then have to help a lot of people at once. Is it not better to let people get up as and when they want to, spreading the demand for staff help?

The major events in Homes are usually mealtimes. Mostly, the days are spent in sitting – sometimes sitting reading, thinking, watching television, or knitting, but more often in sitting doing nothing. This is often difficult to interpret. Some people sit apathetically because of lack of stimulation and general disinterest or depression. Others sit and watch, perhaps taking an interest in the activities of staff, watching the children on their way to and from school, or just watching the squirrels on the lawn. Doing nothing physically does not necessarily mean the mind is inactive.

Mealtimes punctuate the general inactivity with bursts of movement: to and from the toilet and to and from the dining-room. These are times of crowded corridors and doorways. Occasionally some residents will be involved in helping to direct others to their places, settling at tables, serving food, collecting sticks and walking frames. This can be a very positive aspect to their lives.

The routines do not, therefore, affect everyone in the same way. The more frail residents who need more help are least likely to have control of their daily programme: they rely on others to initiate activities. The more able residents are less subject to the influence of rules and routines.

The day is also punctuated by various caring activities and personnel: a visiting chiropodist or physiotherapist, a hospital out-patient appointment, a visit from the community nurse, and especially bathing.

Going to bed usually happens over a more prolonged period than getting up. In Local Authority Homes it is common practice for staff on afternoon and evening shifts to help the majority of people to bed. Only those who are fit enough to put themselves to bed are likely to be up after 10 p.m. when the night staff come on duty. This is not always the case, but it seems to be a predominant pattern. People will be making their way to bed, with or without help, from as early as 7 or 7.30. Most will be on their way after an evening drink or light supper. This can be an important way of setting the pattern. If the supper drink is provided at 7.30, that provokes earlier retiring to bed than if it is served an hour or two later. Of course, the earlier residents go to bed the earlier they are inclined to get up the next morning.

Residents are different from each other: an obvious but too easily forgotten point. They are also different from day to day. The basic principle should be to find out what each person is used to and wants and then to try to provide that. Many have always gone to bed and got up early; some hardly need sleep. In the end, it should be up to them.

Eating and drinking

Food and drink are essentials of survival. They also provide a focus for social interaction.

The way in which meals are served, the elements of choice and the degree of control an individual resident can exercise are important elements. Mealtimes are one way in which routines can control life-style for the whole group. They can be hurried, unsociable occasions. Since they are such an important feature of daily routine and one of the most central occasions for talking to others, they are an opportunity for a more leisurely, social occasion. They should offer time for people to relax, enjoy the food and to talk to each other. Food needs to be well presented and served appropriately: if there are tureens and teapots, then residents will have cause to ask for and give help. Yes, some residents may be too confused to eat in an acceptable manner but that needs to be managed individually and cannot be a reason to serve everyone with ready-plated meals, or from a common teapot.

Many Homes now seek to offer a flexible breakfast time from

around 8 a.m., which enables residents to get up when they want and eat when it suits them. Usually, cooked food is available on a more restricted basis. Many Homes do, however, expect all residents to eat breakfast at a fixed time and most will have fixed lunch and evening mealtimes. There is sometimes more flexibility, especially in private Homes: sometimes this is because of restricted dining room space rather than a wish to offer positive choice.

The main meal of the day is usually around midday. A high tea will be provided at about 4 to 4.30 in the afternoon; a light supper of a drink and biscuits or sandwiches is a typical pattern. One consequence of this pattern (often dictated by the arrangement of catering staff rotas) is that residents have their main food intake between 8 a.m. and 5 p.m.: leaving almost two-thirds of the 24 hour period with no substantial food intake.

Again, the guiding principle should be residents' wishes. We know, however, that if we ask a group of residents what they want they are inclined to express a preference for what already happens. Finding out what they would really prefer may be a lengthy process of offering choices and experimenting with some different ways of doing it. It is not enough to introduce changes: there must be discussion, consultation, experiment and flexibility. Above all, does it have to be done the same way for everybody?

Bathing

Most people bathe in the morning or in the evening. Most elderly residents find themselves being offered a bath during the day. That is when staff are available to help: most residents get help with bathing and staff believe that it is unacceptably risky to leave them to bathe alone.

Bathing during the day means undressing and dressing again. It involves extra staff time and is tiring for residents.

Those who choose not to bathe may be subjected to a variety of pressures from encouragement to bullying or being labelled as uncooperative. But good health and hygiene do not *necessarily* require routine immersion in water. Is there not room to treat people differently, according to their wishes?

The social environment: some key questions

Being 'resident-orientated'

- Do routines meet staff needs or resident needs first?
- Can residents choose to be different or are they all treated the same?
- Do the more frail residents have the same opportunities as the more able?

Being respectful

- Are residents spoken to with respect?
- What are residents called? Is it how they have chosen to be addressed?
- Do staff speak to residents in a manner which is appropriate for people of their age?

Tolerating reasonable and responsible risk-taking

- Are there any limitations on residents going out? When they want to? Alone?
- Can residents bathe unsupervised if they wish?

PEOPLE AND RELATIONSHIPS: SETTING SOME OBJECTIVES

To conclude this discussion of the basic elements of what Homes actually do, some issues and further principles can be highlighted.

Setting goals

For all sorts of reasons, staff should have a clear idea of what they want to achieve. They need to know in order to check on their progress, to provide training to others and to share their objectives with residents.

One way of clarifying goals is by the development of a brochure for the Home. *Home Life* (Centre for Policy on Ageing 1984) advocates a brochure which should set out the aims of the management, including:

- the type of resident catered for;
- the degree of care offered;

- the extent to which illness and disability can be accommodated;
- any restrictions relating to age, sex, religion, etc.

It should also describe the facilities, staffing and accommodation and should include a clear statement of the terms under which the accommodation is offered, including:

- the level of fees and when and how to pay and the procedure for increasing fees;
- the services covered by fees and any services charged separately;
- terms on which a resident may be temporarily away from the Home;
- circumstances in which she might be asked to leave;
- procedures for making a complaint;
- procedure on the death of a resident.

Such a brochure is equally appropriate for both Local Authority and independent-sector Homes. It should be available before application to the Home.

A brochure can set out general aims and objectives. The more detailed goals for staff (e.g. to wash curtains in the next month; or to establish a key worker system) may need to be set out and reviewed more frequently. This may be done at staff meetings or at an annual unit review which can take an overview of all current resources and activities in the Home.

Goals may be set for each resident through a system of care plans: this is discussed in more detail later (see pp. 132–9).

Whatever the goals, if they are to be successfully implemented it is essential that:

- they are known to the people who have to implement them;
- those who are to carry them out should understand and be committed to them: they therefore have to be realistic and related to what people believe;
- everyone should understand who is responsible for doing what;
- they should be capable of amendment if circumstances should change.

Seeing people as individuals

This discussion has put a lot of emphasis on the differences between people: on treating them individually. This begins with recognizing their unique value and experiences: 80 or 90 years of life must have included a great deal of problem-solving and valuable learning. We should start with that recognition, with understanding who and what people have been and valuing their skills and knowledge. At its simplest this involves calling them by the name they choose to use – not calling everyone by first names without their permission (and the fact that they do not protest is not necessarily 'permission').

The follow-on from this is the importance of listening to what the residents as a whole want. Consulting with consumers and responding to their opinions is an essential part of any good service delivery.

Many Homes have experimented with Residents' committees and with other ways of enabling residents to take part in decision-making. Mixed success is reported. This is sometimes related to the abilities of one or two able and articulate residents who make a committee work through force of personality. Sometimes success is related to the skills and commitment of staff. Skills of helping groups to work effectively are an essential part of residential work, as later discussion will show. Effective use of groups is related to the ability of leaders to recognize the individual contribution of each person to the overall pattern of group behaviour.

Creating a total environment

At the opposite end of the spectrum, the residential worker has to be concerned with the whole environment of the Home. The worker must, therefore, be able to find the balance of individual needs and responses with attention to the whole.

This discussion has ranged over a variety of tasks and principles. To summarize, there are probably three main perspectives to keep in mind.

1 A homely environment

A large institution has some unavoidable problem features. In particular, it restricts residents and tends to cut them off from outside contacts, limiting the choices they can make because of the needs of the larger group.

A Home cannot, therefore, be truly homely in a domestic sense. It can, however, offer some of the features of home that people most value: warmth, security, comfort and a degree of control over the immediate personal environment.

2 An enabling environment

Homes have the potential to offer rehabilitation by enabling people to learn or relearn skills to do things for themselves.

Routines are often built up around the needs of staff to carry out a lot of tasks in a short time for many people. Staff often find it easier and quicker to do things to or for people rather than with them. Skills are underused and may be lost simply because *too much* care is provided.

A good Home will be one in which residents are enabled to perform independently all those things they want to do for themselves.

There is also a specific sense in which a Home can be created as a healing and enabling environment through the use of colour, decoration and furnishing which enhance feelings of well-being and encourage self-care.

3 A safe environment

Residents say they value security. Protection can, however, be restricting.

It will never be possible to make Homes absolutely safe in the sense of being completely free of hazards. They can be made to be reasonably safe in the sense that hazards are kept to a minimum in a building with the best possible design and materials to reduce risk. Risk-taking has been identified as an essential and even desirable part of residential living. A resident should be able to choose her own risks, just as anyone else would.

Anyone choosing to drive at speed on a busy road would take precautions to ensure that brakes and steering are in good condition and would expect the road to be well maintained, and would hope other road users would drive sensibly. In the same way, residential Homes should provide an environment which is reasonably and realistically safe and within which responsible behaviour will ensure protection without too much intrusion into the quality of life.

WHAT DO HOMES DO? SUMMARY OF KEY ISSUES

This chapter set out to *describe* what Homes do, what they are like in day-to-day practice, and to establish some of the key principles of good practice and their practical implications. Particularly important elements of this are:

- Residential Homes are *institutions* and as such share some features in common with other institutions such as prisons or hospitals. These features have generally been described critically: loss of liberty and autonomy, experience of social stigma, depersonalization – all in the context of poor material standards.
- The atmosphere, overall life-style or *regime* of a Home can be understood in a total sense of a 'good' or a 'bad' Home, but also in terms of some specific dimensions: the physical environment, the people who live and work in it, their interactions with each other and the rules and routines of social behaviour. There are many professional prescriptions about how to create a good life-style but the research evidence that these actually affect resident dependency or functional ability is scarce and confusing.
- To understand and measure the standard of care it is necessary to distinguish between *quality of care* (such as things that are provided for residents, the physical environment and staff behaviour) and *quality of life* as the experience of each resident (or consumer satisfaction). There are some things which do seem to be related to residents' satisfaction: freedom from worry; feeling comfortable; being able to control the immediate environment; and the company of chosen companions.
- Creating a good Home involves ensuring that there is a 'fit' or congruence between what people want and are able to deal with and the pressures and potentials of their environment. The environment can be seen as made up of *physical features,* the *social environment* of rules and routines and the *people and relationships* available. Each of these dimensions needs to be

considered and developed in setting and achieving goals for the Home as a whole and for each individual in it.

WHERE TO LEARN MORE

Useful, relatively short books which discuss design issues are:

Norman, A. (1984) *Bricks and Mortals*, London: Centre for Policy on Ageing.
Peace, S.M.(1982) *A Balanced Life? A Consumer Study of Residential Life in a Hundred Local Authority Old People's Homes*, Polytechnic of North London.

Jones and Fowles (1984) offer the best introduction to ideas about institutions and Booth (1985) covers a range of issues about regimes.

A particularly thorough review of the literature up to 1980 can be found in:

Davies, B. and Knapp, M. (1981) *Old People's Homes and the Production of Welfare*, London: Routledge & Kegan Paul.

A more recent research-based discussion of residential life is

Willcocks, D. *et al.* (1987) *Private Lives in Public Places*, London: Tavistock Publications.

Finally, it would be useful to dip into a collection of papers, referred to in the text, presented to a DHSS seminar on Residential Care for the Elderly in October 1983 (Judge and Sinclair 1986)

Chapter Five

GATEKEEPING: PROCESSES OF ADMISSION AND ASSESSMENT

The nature of residential Homes is very much dependent on the people who live in them. The care needed and the life-style that results will be influenced by the types of people who come in and the demands they make.

The decisions made about who comes in and how they get there are therefore very important. The person who controls access – the gatekeeper – holds great power.

This chapter will therefore look at some of the decision-making processes, the reasons why elderly people go into Homes, the actual processes of moving in and the effects of going in. These will be linked to what we know about how to ease the transition and help people to move on and develop. Finally, there will be a discussion of the processes of making assessments and reviewing the needs of individuals before, during and after admission.

COMING IN: THE ADMISSION PROCESS

The phrase 'admission to care' itself raises some interesting questions. The commonly used word 'admission' seems to imply some use of power or authority: someone permits, allows or even compels the elderly person to enter a Home.

Before proceeding to consider the evidence about elderly people it will be worth spending some time considering the process of admission more generally. Much of the material that has been written about the admission process has been relatively short and devoted to specific situations or client groups. Until recently, little attention has been given to the common elements in the process; yet some common elements do exist and offer a basis for the elaboration of more specific discussion of how to take action.

One difficulty has been in clarifying the nature of 'care', which is a word that has been used in many different contexts with a wide range of meanings. Care describes the way people feel about others but it also describes things done to or for them. Admission to care is not a single concept or process: it might, perhaps, be defined as moving from living in a family or community environment to a protected and/or restricted environment. But such a view does not cover all the possibilities satisfactorily. A Care Order on a child, for instance, permits the child to be returned home to his family and, in this sense, the entry into the status 'in care' does not involve environmental change. There is an important distinction between the change of status involved in admission (which may involve change of legal status or simply change of role, e.g. from householder to resident) and the change of environment. People may feel differently about these different kinds of changes.

It has been extensively argued that admission to care is a process which involves distinct, recognizable stages. Nevertheless, the complexity of the background to admission – the organizational context, the people involved, the legal and professional background, the language used – means the actual experience (how it feels and what actually happens) varies widely between individuals.

Perhaps the most comprehensive attempt to identify stages in the process was by Jones (1972) who used a broad framework of separation/transition/incorporation to break down the admission process into 24 stages. She argued, through the comparison of practical examples, that situations as unalike as a confused old lady entering a psychiatric hospital and a divorced stockbroker planning a holiday in Cannes, have common process elements. Pope (1978) slightly extended these elements into four stages which he called preparation, separation, transition and incorporation. These four stages provide a useful basis for discussing good practice in admitting elderly people to care. They must be seen within various perspectives: of decision-making; of economic or administrative pressures; of socialization and initiation into the new Home; of differing time-scales; and, above all, in relation to the meaning of the experience to the individual who is living through it.

The admission process has most often been described in gloomy terms and it would be easy to produce a list of quotations from writers who have stressed the negative features of care. Many such features have been noted: loss of status; feelings of inadequacy, guilt, anger, powerlessness and shame; the breaking of ties and consequent feelings of loss and guilt; the indignity of being 'processed'; and the implication that the person coming into care has in some way 'failed' in her previous life. Separation, loss and exposure to potentially stressful situations are a feature of many, if not all, admissions, yet there is a more positive dimension. The admission process does bring benefits and foremost of these must be the sanctuary which a protected environment offers. There is an important distinction between preventing admission to care and preventing deprivation. Residential care may be regarded as second best by almost everyone; however, there are many occasions when to admit to care may be hazardous but not to do so may be even more so.

This leads to another important factor: residential care is primarily used as a resource to manage risk. People of all ages go into different forms of care because they are exposed to a wide variety of risks. In other words, they are exposed to recognizable hazards and are therefore judged to be 'in danger' in their current living situation. In this sense residential care aims to provide an environment which is safer than the previous home situation. This is a fairly limited view as there is ample evidence that leaving a familiar environment and entering a strange, unfamiliar situation carries with it a new set of risks, both physical and emotional. In addition, life in an enclosed residential Home involves exposure to a further set of risks which have also been well documented (although it should be remembered that risk-taking is increasingly accepted as a necessary feature of good residential life: this is discussed later in more detail).

Admission to care is not a step to be taken lightly: it should only be pursued if it is clear that the likely benefits of admission outweigh the potential disadvantages. Unfortunately our ability to predict these sorts of outcomes is very limited.

WHAT KIND OF PROCESS IS ADMISSION?

One perspective focuses on residential care as a *helping resource*, and admission is primarily seen in terms of the most efficient and effective use of the resource.

Another widely discussed view presents admission as *an experience of crisis*. Berry (1972) has argued, for instance, that the client coming into care comes from a state of crisis and also that the admission is itself a crisis. The fact that admission has been judged necessary may be an indication that the client has failed to adapt to an earlier crisis and the fact that she has failed (or believes she has failed) before is likely to make it more difficult for her to manage the new crisis presented by admission. Admission to care may, in other words, be a stressful experience made more stressful by the feelings of loss and distress which the client brings with her from the situation which led to the need for admission. The implications for action seem to be the importance of helping people during the transition from one environment to another with their feelings about the move, as well as with the practicalities of moving, in order to encourage a positive adaptation to the changes.

A further important element in discussion of the admission process has been the stress which has often been placed on entry to care as *an experience of separation*. The literature on the impact of separation on children and their parents is well known and does not require elaboration here. It is now widely accepted that it is the existence of close emotional ties or bonds between the child and an attachment figure which is important to healthy development in the long term. Such findings are clearly important to the social worker admitting a child to care. It is less clear how far these assumptions can be transferred to adults. It is likely that admission to care will often be distressing and will represent separation from important friends and relatives for many elderly residents. Whether or not the distress will have a lasting effect and the extent to which the elderly person will be able to make positive use of the residential facilities and enjoy life will certainly be affected by how the distress is handled. Both field and residential workers have an important role in helping to keep stress and distress to a minimum.

Separation is, of course, a two-sided experience and often too little consideration is given to those who are left behind. In one sense, those left at home may need help in their own right with feelings of guilt or loss or help with material and physical or other emotional difficulties. In another sense it is important to work with them because of the need to keep open the possibility of an escape route for the elderly person who may wish to return at some stage.

Admission to care is also for some people *an experience of compulsion*. There is an obvious and fundamental difference between receiving people into care in the sense that they come voluntarily, without the use of legal authority, and removing people from home for care, treatment or containment with the use of formal, legal authority. Between these two ends of the continuum lies a large area of uncertainty. Pressure from relatives, neighbours, doctors and social workers is frequently considerable. Although the vast majority of admissions are made without the use of statutory authority it seems likely that many are the result of less formal but none the less real compulsion or 'persuasion'. Although the process of admission – involving beginning, middle and end phases – is similar whether or not there is compulsion, the element of authority is an important determinant of the nature and extent of social work involvement in the process.

Similarly, the fact that some admissions are carried out in a hurry does not necessarily alter the nature of the stages of the admission process. But it will have an important effect on the kinds of social work involvement. The time dimension is one more important variable in the process. Many admissions are called emergencies. It is important to distinguish between the true emergency situation, when admission may be the only way to avoid serious danger, loss or damage, and the panic situation in which there is subjective pressure to act in a hurry but in which the objective needs and risks are actually less pressing. The danger in the latter case is that the admission process will be inadequately carried out and the opportunity to make the most effective use of the potentials of residential care may be lost.

Admission to care can, then, be seen as a process involving a series of distinct events: recognizing something is wrong or likely to go wrong, deciding to take action, preparation and the actual move from one place to another; and, finally, arriving and settling in. The decisions and approaches within the process will be affected by many factors and the time taken and emphasis on each stage will vary.

It has also been suggested here that admission can be thought of in terms of its perspectives as a resource, as an experience of loss and separation and as an experience, potentially, of compulsion, crisis or emergency. Any discussion or description of 'good practice' in admission to care can draw from these common assumptions, but any generalized statement about what kinds of actions are good or bad when admitting elderly people to Homes will need a great deal of qualification and involves some complex value assumptions.

Two particular messages from this discussion are important. In the first place, admission is risky: existing crisis, compounded by separation and loss, compulsion and environmental change, creates its own dangers. The hazards of the process can be identified and the possibilities for taking action to avoid, minimize, or remove them weighed up. In the second place, admission is a process of change through time which will be experienced differently by the different people involved: it is the way people perceive things, how they feel about what is happening to them, that is really important.

WHY DO ELDERLY PEOPLE COME INTO HOMES?

Chapter 2 reviewed some of the more common difficulties that affect elderly people. The majority do express themselves to be satisfied with their lives: many of them are more satisfied than younger people, in spite of being in objectively worse circumstances. However, a substantial minority, perhaps around one in five, are very dissatisfied. This is usually related in particular to greater age, ill health and the quality of relationships with family and friends. More than anything, it is the 'cluster of circumstances', the collecting together of a group of problems and difficulties which as a whole are beyond the coping capacity of the elderly individual.

Most commonly, residents have been living alone immediately before coming in. This is even more the case for women. About one in five have been living with relatives and about a quarter in another institution, most commonly a hospital, before admission. Men are more likely than women to have been living with a spouse before coming in.

This pattern has been changing over time. The tendency is increasingly for people to have been living alone in the community before admission. Fewer have been living with a relative. This is no doubt a reflection of changing patterns of community services and expectations of caring relatives but is also related to changes in age structure of the population (Lawrence *et al.* 1987).

The reasons for seeking a place in a Home fall into four broad, interlinked groups:

1 Inability to manage personal care: they cannot look after themselves. Studies of age and dependency have varied in their findings. It has been suggested that, as a rough guide, in a typical study around 20 in every 100 residents will be less than 73 years old. Forty will be between 75 and 84 and the remaining 40 will be 85 or over. The average in all studies is high: around 82 to 83 years amongst residents and a year or so less amongst applicants (Sinclair 1986). Some applicants are severely disabled. The majority are not but do have specific difficulties in carrying out certain tasks such as those necessary to cooking a hot meal or making a hot drink.
2 Exposure to hazards: being at risk. Quite simply, Local Authority criteria for applications are usually couched in terms of risk: the elderly person must be at risk in their usual home circumstances before they can be considered. The picture that emerges is that the majority of applicants for Homes are very old, physically and mentally frail and socially unsupported. Health reasons and the need for surveillance – someone to keep an eye on their safety – often figure large in reasons given. This is complex. Illness is different from disability which is itself a difficult concept: there is a difference between the physical effects of a disease process and the things those effects prevent people from doing: the social and personal care tasks they can no longer carry out. It is, however, clear that physical 'dis-eases' and mental infirmity play a large part in application decisions.
3 The burden on carers: an elderly person's right to stay at home may in practice depend on her daughter's willingness

101

and ability to continue providing time, support and practical help. Since many people considering entering care now do so when they are aged over 80 it is common to find they are being cared for by children who are themselves approaching or past retirement age. The choice of whether to enter care or not is therefore not simply about the hazards to the elderly person but also about the hazards to health and happiness which that decision may create for their family. Similarly, the caring professional or voluntary worker providing support during the decision is faced with a number of dilemmas in balancing the various needs and wishes. To support the elderly person in a decision to remain at home carries the risk of, for instance, blame or guilt if that person should die alone or in distress. Deciding whether or not to enter a Home involves taking risks, not least of which is the danger to the helper of feeling responsible and being held responsible for a wrong decision.

4 Precipitating factors: many requests for admission present themselves as emergencies. Sudden events such as bereavement, loss of a carer, or a fall or other crisis illness can often make the difference between coping and not coping and precipitate a decision to apply for a place in a Home. More importantly, such an event can be the justification for offering a place to one elderly person in preference to others in otherwise similar circumstances. There are, however, signs that the growth of private care is affecting the pressure on beds, in combination with changes and developments in the use of home care and other domiciliary services. There may, therefore, be less pressure to provide permanent care in response to crisis and to offer short-term care and respite whilst the elderly person gains the strength to make a more considered decision.

There is conflicting evidence about whether those who go into Homes need to do so. In the first place there is an argument that no-one needs residential care and that all could be provided for if community services were extensive and flexible enough. But it has also been suggested that a proportion of admissions are unnecessary in the sense that they result from inadequate medical assessment: it is argued that a full medical assessment and treatment could lead to improved coping capacities and remove the need for care for some people.

In spite of changes and innovations in the use of community services in more imaginative and creative 'packages of care' to keep people in their own homes, social workers are reported to believe that between one- and two-thirds of those admitted to residential care could be maintained in the community if there were appropriate services (National Institute for Social Work 1988). Other evidence from the private sector (Gibbs and Bradshaw 1987b) suggests that the vast majority (over 90 per cent) of people in Homes are in need of residential care at the time of admission. A small proportion of these (some 2 per cent) were felt to have recovered sufficiently to be able to leave the Home. An important finding of this study was that virtually all those admitted from hospital were judged to be appropriately placed, whereas around 11 per cent of those admitted from the community were judged to be misplaced.

There is ample evidence that a high proportion of people going into Homes do so reluctantly. Some do choose to go in, but the majority see it as the 'least unpleasant' choice rather than the best. This has important implications for how they adjust to life in the Home. New arrangements for assessment before the Local Authority agrees to provide care, following the Community Care White Paper (Department of Health, 1989), may have an important effect on choice.

MAKING DECISIONS

Many factors will be involved in the decision of the elderly person to apply for a place in a Home on a permanent basis. Often the decision will not be freely made and will have been subject to a combination of pressures from family, neighbours and professionals or the practical constraints of an unsuitable environment.

Most applications for Homes will in future be subject to assessment by social workers and their managers. Residential workers are less likely to have an influence. There is, as was shown earlier, evidence that social work with elderly people has low status. It is often not central to their social care: often because the doubts people have about the effectiveness of social workers lead to a bypassing of them to the more practical sources of help, such as home-care services.

Social work help is primarily short term and is practically focused. Elderly clients and their carers are often satisfied with the help they get: particularly where that help is practical. Short-term involvement of Social Services Department social workers will often involve qualified workers, although much of the longer-term work is done by unqualified social work assistants. Field social workers can have a key role in helping elderly people who need substantial amounts of social and personal care support. It is generally agreed that their role should include assessment, mobilizing resources and managing individual packages of care, and providing information, advice, counselling and support to elderly people and their carers.

There is no doubt that social workers have had a pivotal role in decisions about Local Authority Homes. The picture has been more complicated in the independent sector: evidence is scarce, the picture has changed rapidly, and will do so again as new assessment arrangements by the Local Authorities develop for people going into all Homes, following the 1989 White Paper. The attitudes of local Councils to the involvement of social workers in advising and guiding people about suitable places in the private sector have varied. Few will do more than provide a list of Homes, with little guidance on the quality of what is available. Often hospital social workers have a central role in helping people find a private Home and there is evidence that people admitted from hospital are rather more likely to be appropriately placed than those coming from the community.

Around one-third of people applying for Local Authority places do so from hospital. Once in hospital the pressures on an elderly person to make and stick to a decision to apply for a place in a Home can be quite considerable. Yet it has often been suggested that a proportion of admissions to Homes are unnecessary. A number of studies have shown that a high proportion of people going into Homes have treatable illnesses whose effects could be reduced or minimized. Full assessments, including medical input are relatively rare, especially for people coming from the community rather than from hospital.

There are strong arguments for improving multi-disciplinary approaches to assessment. There is particular concern that those

elderly people who go into private Homes will have less opportunity for a full review of their needs and the options open to them.
The evidence for this is, however, limited. Medical screening can,
however, delay admission to residential care and open up alternative options, such as sheltered housing.

Many people come into Homes in a hurry. There is pressure for
urgent action and little time for full assessment. The emphasis on
emergency may be the result of the fact that many do not ask for
help until they are forced to do so. It may be because resources are
limited and only those who can show they are in greatest need can
get in. It may also be that screening and preventive social work are
less effective than they might be. Whatever the reasons, the haste
with which many admissions are arranged does create problems.

The bad news . . .

- Many people apply for Homes with very little information
  about what to expect. If they are to make an informed
  decision from amongst choices, they must have knowledge of
  what those options are.
- Most apply at a time when they are least able to make an
  informed choice. Usually, people seek to go into residential
  care as a last resort and are in crisis, often subject to ill health
  or disability.
- Those coming into residential Homes are, by operational
  definition, a particularly vulnerable group. Many are severely
  disabled. Most have some major difficulties in carrying out
  personal care tasks. A high proportion have a substantial
  degree of mental impairment. They come from crisis and
  situations of high risk but are actually the group who are most
  vulnerable to the stress of moving: the least likely to survive
  change.
- It has been extensively argued that going into residential care
  leads to deterioration and death. The evidence is
  complicated: it seems clear that some people are especially
  vulnerable to the effects of moving from one place to another
  and may deteriorate or die in consequence. The factors that
  influence this are probably the strengths and weaknesses of
  the person moving, the preparations for the move, and the
  quality of the environment they are moving to. The most
  important point is that moving elderly people from one place

to another is stressful and can be dangerous, even to the extent of introducing the risk of death for some.

- Entry to a Home can also have negative psychological effects. Elderly people come from difficult situations and will feel grief for the loss of their home and all that it meant to them. They are then exposed to a large group of others whom they may see as sick, dependent, mentally infirm and apathetic. One danger is that they may identify with this group and fall into similar patterns of behaviour, simply because that seems to be the way to behave in that particular place.

- Some evidence suggests that the typical behaviour of someone in long-term institutional care is actually traceable to the period before admission and is linked to the decision to apply. This may be linked to feelings of loss, separation and abandonment (Tobin and Lieberman 1976). It becomes a period of preparatory withdrawal.

But the good news . . .

- Those who feel they have made a free choice to move are less likely to feel unhappy or to suffer physical deterioration after admission.

- Feeling in control of the decision is linked to having information about choices. If there is good information and careful planning some of the main stresses can be reduced.

- The degree of change involved is a significant element. If the new environment is similar to the former, then the stresses are fewer. This is often difficult to arrange but some simple things – like bringing in furniture, photographs and other personal possessions – can assist with continuity. Maintaining familiar links with friends or day centres for a time will also help some.

- Efficient arrangements for the move are also important. Making sure that everything is ready beforehand, that cars are on time and that someone is on hand to greet the new arrival at the Home are simple but essential elements in reducing the stress.

- One of the most important factors in a successful move is the experience and ability of each person to cope: if she has always been able to cope with change then she is more likely to settle in successfully.

A brief checklist of factors should be borne in mind:

1 Moving from one place to another can be dangerous: it exposes elderly people to emotional and physical stress and infections, etc. Just moving is itself potentially stressful.
2 Deciding to apply for a Home can be a trigger to withdrawn and self-centred behaviour. People waiting for care can feel abandoned and depressed at the anticipation of loss and change.
3 Those with physical ill health and/or mental infirmity are especially vulnerable: on the whole, those who go into Homes are those most likely to be damaged as a result!
4 Those who have always been passive in their approach to life are less likely to make a 'successful adjustment'. Demanding, hostile or 'pushy' behaviour can actually be a good indication of likely survival.
5 Feeling rejected is associated with unsuccessful admissions: on the other hand, those who feel they have freely chosen to move are more likely to settle.
6 Careful planning and preparation for the move reduce stress.
7 The more moderate the change of environment, the less marked the effect may be: contact and links with the previous life are important.
8 The quality of the new environment (the Home) is a major factor.

THE RESIDENTIAL WORKER'S ROLE IN ADMISSION: GETTING IT RIGHT

There may be practical differences between the private and Local Authority settings but the basic principles will be the same in each. Central aspects will be: information and choice; making the move; settling in; handling emergencies; and hospital transfers.

Information and choice

Residential workers have a part to play in making sure that potential applicants know what they could expect: what they can expect whilst their application is being considered and after admission. They can contribute by:

- Providing written information. This can be done effectively through a brochure designed to answer the most common questions applicants ask.
- Visiting the applicant's own home. This helps to make a link for the elderly person but enables residential staff to see and understand more about the applicant's previous life and achievements.
- Enabling the applicant to visit the Home to meet staff and talk at leisure to other residents. Sometimes this can only be a brief visit. A full day is desirable and it is increasingly common for people to stay for at least one period of a week or so to get used to the Home. There is strong support from research for such a considered approach for most people.
- Being involved in case conferences and admission decisions. Field social workers often make decisions about admissions without themselves having more than a superficial knowledge of the Home they are deciding about. Residential staff involvement is an essential element.
- Ensuring that the staff in the Home know who is coming and have essential information about that person. Assessment is considered later but 'essential' information will be enough to ensure that daily needs are properly met, as well as enough to enable staff to develop a proper respect for the skills and life experience of that resident.

Making the move

The detailed arrangements for giving up the home and the actual day of the move will often be made by a field social worker or family. The residential worker can contribute by:

- Making clear to the resident, family or social worker what is expected and needed. A simple checklist of things to think about, from reading the gas meter to the packing of towels, will be useful.
- Making sure someone meets and has time to give to the new arrival. It is relatively easy to make the practical preparations: the room should be ready, a cup of tea waiting, time available to help unpack, etc.
- Helping to make contact with existing residents. This is more

difficult and is discussed in greater detail later. First contact with one or two friendly residents and guidance on where to sit, where to eat and the basic routines will help avoid immediate difficulties.

Settling in

Opinions differ on how long the settling-in period lasts. Some suggest that after a month or so the resident will have found a pace and pattern to life. Others argue that the stresses and strains of admission extend for at least two or three months. I think people react differently!

Residential workers can help by:

- Ensuring that one member of staff is responsible for frequent personal contact with the new resident and for finding a quiet time regularly to talk to her.
- Encouraging family, friends and social worker to keep in close touch to maintain continuity and reduce feelings of abandonment. There is, of course, a fine balance: too many contacts may be unsettling.
- Planning a regular review of how things are going, including family, social worker, doctor, nurse, etc., as necessary.

Handling emergencies

In spite of the most careful planning strategies it is a fact that some people come into Homes with limited and inadequate assessment, little information and without having visited the Home before-hand. Those who do so are, by definition, particularly vulnerable because they will have come from crisis. They will need especially sensitive help and support in the settling-in period. The residential worker can help by making sure that the way back is kept open so that the elderly person can return home if she is able to recover in the secure environment of the Home.

Hospital transfers

A substantial proportion of admissions are from hospitals and it is important that the transfer is not just treated as an administrative procedure. Links between hospital and residential staff will be valuable in many ways and should be developed at every opportunity. It is unusual now for admissions to be made on a 'swap' basis, but it is important that arrangements are not made in too much of a hurry. The applicant should have a few days to plan and prepare for a move and should have a chance to discuss the future and the same information and opportunities to visit the Home as anyone else. The residential worker may need to take a controlling role in this if it is to be done properly. It is essential that family and friends are kept informed and involved at this stage: they have a part to play in getting the basics right, down to ensuring that teeth, spectacles and hearing-aids are not forgotten and that clothing is appropriate on the day of the move.

In summary

Essential principles are:
- giving full information;
- involving the applicant fully;
- managing the moving day efficiently;
- preparing the Home properly: the room, the staff and the residents;
- maintaining the links with past life as much as possible;
- remembering first impressions are important;
- applying these principles to short, as well as long-stay admissions.

ASSESSMENT AND REVIEW

There is an argument that residential Homes should simply provide a comfortable and homely environment and that to insist on detailed assessments of each individual is to be intrusive and invests a set of everyday tasks with an unnecessary professional mystique. The nature of the assessment needed will probably depend on circumstances. It has earlier been established that most elderly people are in Homes because of physical or mental frailty, disability or some other need for personal assistance from other people. In order to provide help effectively, there is a need for workers to be clear about what help they are able to offer and to apply that to the needs of individuals (match resources with identified need).

This implies an assessment. Assessment is about understanding, describing, measuring, evaluating, deciding; it is a complex activity. Essentially, there are four basic elements to assessment: collecting information; evaluation; making a decision; and taking action.

Collecting information

Information should be *relevant*. It should not be collected simply because it is interesting or because it may be useful someday. It should be useful for a purpose in hand.

It should be *accurate*. This means that we need to have ways of collecting information which are reliable. Good assessment depends on good communication: communication with frail, mentally infirm, elderly people, many of whom suffer from impaired sight or hearing, is likely to be difficult and requires special skills.

It should be *up-to-date*. We need to be sure that what we think we know is still current. It is common to find information on files which has been passed from one worker to another and may well have been inaccurate in the first place, or misunderstood in the passing on, or simply out-of-date.

It should be *confidential*. Residential Homes are particularly difficult places in which to keep private information restricted. Information about a resident should be regarded as belonging to that person and must not be passed to anyone without her permission or unless there is very good reason to do so. At a basic level, this requires decisions to be made and clearly understood about who has access to personal files.

It should be *available to the person concerned*, within limits. There are legal rules about how records should be made available and about the restrictions that may be placed on some kinds of information. The best way to make sure that information is accurate and up-to-date is to share what is written down with the resident concerned. In some Homes residents hold their own files as a record of their experience. This is a good way of achieving accuracy, relevance and involvement.

Evaluation

Information has to be given meaning before it can be used. The way it is organized will affect the meanings given. Many application forms, for instance, are completed by social workers who tend to stress the negatives: that is how they make a case for admission. The information is therefore about what people cannot do rather than what they can do. Similarly, the way in which the person collecting the information views elderly people may affect the way it is structured and used. It may emphasize the potentials and possibilities; on the other hand, it may focus on the difficulties, limitations and restrictions on elderly people.

Information about a person and her needs becomes an 'assessment of need' when it is related to some possible goal or service. 'She is lonely' thus becomes 'she needs company'; 'she is ill' becomes 'she needs medicine'. 'Need' is a difficult word and it may be helpful to explore it in a little more depth. Needs are relative to circumstances and will vary amongst societies, individuals and generations. Although need implies a goal or idea of satisfaction, the same basic need may be satisfied in different ways.

In a collective sense we talk about need in terms of what is generally acceptable as a way of responding to particular problems. 'She needs residential care' is a generally understood and acceptable response to particular types of problems. This is then related to what people can have in a given situation. It may be agreed and accepted that someone needs residential care but she may still not receive that service because it is not available at the time.

Needs may therefore be related to goals and to alternative means of achieving those goals. Needs become specific when goals are defined. But this does not take account of the idea of 'drive': people may have needs of which they are not aware, they may feel needs, and they may have wishes. There is a difference between unfelt need, felt need, and desire.

Need may operate in a negative sense as a push to escape from discomfort. It may also act in a positive sense as a pull towards something that attracts. The aim should perhaps not be to eliminate need but to enable positive need to operate: to relieve deprivation and discomfort and provide people with opportunities for positive drives towards satisfaction to be met in creative ways.

Evaluation therefore has two main elements:

- deciding how to order the information and to give it meaning;
- putting the ordered understanding of a person and her situation together with knowledge about resources, options and goals.

Making a decision

A good assessment must take account of the will and capability of people to define their own needs: to decide what things mean and how they wish to proceed to meet their needs and influence the course of their lives. An assessment is incomplete unless it recognizes the elderly person's definition of the world and that of those close to her. These definitions may, of course, differ: this is not to suggest that the elderly person's definition is in some sense more correct, but that it is at least as important as that of anyone else involved.

An important element in assessment is the interaction between the people involved. By exchanging information and interpretations they influence each other's understanding and perceptions. There is a need, therefore, to provide structured occasions to meet together, share information and discuss possibilities.

Taking action

Once a decision has been made action will usually follow. Assessments should be flexible enough to change and modify if action shows a need to do so. Plans should be *reviewed*.

The process of collecting and ordering information and decision-making is rarely an orderly progression. Elderly people often have a collection of interrelated and complex problems and there are seldom clear-cut solutions. Assessment is therefore a shifting process, requiring backtracking as people change, more is learned and provisions and services develop. In particular, it is essential to set goals which are realistic and achievable.

MAKING AN ASSESSMENT

There are several possible approaches to assessment of elderly people. Some of the more common ways of thinking about it are: the problem balance-sheet; functional assessment; and adaptation.

The problem balance-sheet

This approach tends to list what people can and cannot do. It lists and categorizes, for instance, diseases and social problems. Action to provide help is most likely to be successful where it builds on the strengths. This is most important. Recording of information about elderly people commonly stresses their weaknesses and problems. It rarely records the skills they have developed during a lifetime of work, home-making, child-rearing, etc. We should remember that even today those who reach their eighties are survivors with survival skills which can be used and developed.

One of the most positive approaches to understanding strengths is the biographical approach. By talking to people about their past life we can learn who they are and what they think is important. It can be an effective way of developing respectful relationships for staff to be given the task of building up, with residents, a life history.

Functional assessment

There are many research and practice tools which have been developed to gather and record information about what individual elderly people are able to do. These usually combine three main elements:

- physical abilities to do such things as self-care tasks (washing, dressing, feeding, etc.) or mobility (climbing stairs, walking unaided, etc.);
- intellectual ability to understand information and remember;
- social functioning: the way in which people behave amongst others (sociable, demanding, aggressive, amenable, etc.).

This approach to collecting information is helpful if it is used in conjunction with a more holistic view of people: with a concern for their total needs and life-style. People are not just the sum of their physical and intellectual abilities, although quite minor elements of these can have major effects on the quality of overall life-style. To put it at a basic level, haemorrhoids may have an overriding effect on happiness and relationships with others!

To understand individual needs, therefore, we need both a functional assessment (what can they do?) and a holistic assessment (what is their quality of life?). But we also need to look at them together (what would improve the quality of life and what strengths can we build on to achieve this?).

Adaptation

A central factor in quality-of-life assessment is the relationship between needs and wishes and the environment and resources available to meet them. Satisfaction is basically about what people want and what they can have.

To understand the total situation of an elderly person, therefore, we need to look at them and their needs in relation to the Home and what it has to offer. The assessment of each individual should, in other words, include assessment of the Home itself and what it is able to do for people. This implies a need for flexibility and self-review by residential staff on a routine basis as well as clear goals and objectives for the Home.

People should also be given a chance to operate in a variety of situations and roles to demonstrate their range of abilities. The fact that a resident finds it difficult to cope in one situation does not mean she cannot cope in others. They should be given different chances to do tasks, to meet different people and to use other facilities. In this way they not only get to show what they can do, but they also have more opportunity to find something they want to do.

WHO SHOULD BE INVOLVED IN ASSESSMENT?

Much has been written about the importance of multi-disciplinary assessment. Sometimes it is not made clear what or who this is intended to include. In a residential Home, people with an interest in or commitment to one resident might include, at least:

Head of Home
Care staff/key worker
Cook
Domestic staff
Field social worker
GP
Psychiatrist
Geriatrician
Community nurse
Community psychiatric nurse

Occupational therapist
Physiotherapist
Speech therapist
Chiropodist
Further education tutor
Craft teacher
Resident
Relatives
Friends
Advocates

A list like this makes it obvious that there cannot be a routine, detailed assessment and review of all residents including all of this group. There should, however, be a core group of people with a duty to meet routinely and regularly to consider whether the Home is providing for each individual resident the most effective and satisfying environment possible. This core group might properly include head of Home, social workers, GP, and nurse and be convened by a nominated key worker. Others should be involved as appropriate and special meetings might need to be called as necessary.

There is little opportunity for most professionals to be involved in multi-disciplinary education. There is plenty of evidence that many elderly people going into Homes have substantial amounts of treatable illness. Working together with doctors, nurses and therapists is essential to provide the best possible life-style for elderly residents. It is all too easy to attribute things to 'just old age'. People do not become ill because they are old. They may be disabled by a number of physical impairments as they grow older. Illnesses can be treated and disability reduced by proper therapy – but only if recognized early enough.

The resident and relatives should be involved in discussions to check regularly that there is no major change in circumstances, to ensure that they are fully informed and to be sure that things are going the way they want, as far as is possible.

SO WHAT IS AN ASSESSMENT?

An assessment is a critical and systematic look at an individual's needs within her current environment. It involves:

- getting the relevant people together, including health care professionals;
- establishing the resident's own priorities;
- setting needs and priorities against the potentials and limitations of the Home;
- looking for other resources or more creative ways of using existing resources to meet needs if necessary;
- setting goals which are realistic and achievable within a time-scale which is meaningful for the resident;
- making a plan for each resident which includes an appreciation of strengths as well as weaknesses, and of what she can do as well as what she cannot do;
- monitoring the plan and reviewing it as necessary and at least once every six months.

Particularly important in this process are:

- the paramount importance of good communication;
- the involvement of the resident;
- clear and accurate records;
- the personal qualities, education and commitment of the key worker.

MOVING ON

Getting into Homes in the right way is important, as is making sure that residents' needs are properly assessed and met. But there are other dimensions. The majority of admissions are now for short periods. The need for a planned and supportive approach to those admissions is clear: some of the differences in expectations and needs are considered elsewhere in this book. Some people come in expecting to stay but find they do not like it, or alternatives emerge unexpectedly, or some residents may improve with good care. Whatever the reasons, some do wish to move on.

Most elderly people in residential care are very old and frail and have arrived there in stressful circumstances. It is unrealistic to expect the majority to move on, given current resources and the expectations with which they go in.

There is, however, reason to believe that some people in Homes do have sufficient skills and abilities to be able to cope in a less protected and restricted environment and that some of them want to do so. Sometimes they do not make any move because they are not told of alternatives or given help to seek them out. It is probably unfair to raise the hopes of someone who has gone in expecting to stay, unless there are very clear and available alternatives. It is, however, possible to help some people to move in for short periods to enable them to recover or improve skills, health and strength with a view to moving on.

The options are fairly limited. It is much more difficult and expensive to create a package of care and support in the community from scratch for someone coming out of a Home than it is to build up supports for someone already in the community. There are, however, some possibilities: the growth of very sheltered housing, increasing provision of 'substitute family' placements for some people and using various ordinary housing options with extra care support, even the use of former staff housing attached to some Local Authority Homes to provide a sheltered but less institutional option.

Recent research evidence and practical social work knowledge suggest that moving from an institutional environment to a more independent situation will be most appropriately managed in purpose-designed, small housing units with a package of interwoven services. The safest support system is the one which relies on more than one carer: collapse of caring systems is commonly the result of one person being left to carry the main burden alone.

Three factors seem to be of central importance if elderly people are to be able to move on from residential Homes:

1 The need for planning and assessment from as early in the process of admission as possible: people should go in with some expectation and hope of moving on where there is a realistic prospect of doing so.
2 The importance of continuing review and involvement of the elderly person in decision-making.
3 Carefully constructing detailed plans for leaving and for support after the move which maintains a sense and reality of continuity in the life of the elderly person.

As a final note, it should be remembered that most people die in the Home to which they are admitted. Residential workers must help them to plan and prepare for moving on through death, by discussion, counselling when necessary and practical help. This is considered more fully later.

ADMISSION AND ASSESSMENT: KEY POINTS

This chapter has explored some of the processes of the residential experience, especially coming in, moving on and the importance of assessment and review and of ensuring that residents get the best possible quality of life:

- Admission to any kind of institutional situation exposes people to risks. Often they go in at a time of crisis and experience loss and separation from important people and things in their lives. Usually they also go through a change in status and often this is complicated by the need for compulsion or the need for haste.
- Elderly people come into Homes for a wide range of reasons. The main reasons can be grouped as: the inability to manage personal care; the exposure to hazards and dangers; the burden on carers; and the effects of unexpected precipitating factors.
- Entering residential care exposes elderly people to some specific risks: physical risks of infection and deterioration or even death, and psychological and emotional stress. Some people who go into Homes die because of the move: those who go into a Home are amongst the most vulnerable to its negative effects.
- Good preparation and clear information can help to ease the stress and reduce the risks. Those who feel they have freely made the choice to move are more likely to adapt successfully to the Home.
- Efficient arrangements for the move into the Home and encouragement of links with the past to provide continuity will also help good adaptation.
- Assessment and review are important elements of providing appropriate care to each individual. Assessment is a process of collecting information and evaluating that information in order to make a decision *with* the elderly person and to take action.

- Assessment should include an overall perspective on the quality of life of the individual but also an evaluation of specific aspects of an individual's strengths and abilities within the Home environment. The Home should be flexible in adapting to individual needs.
- There is substantial evidence of treatable illness amongst elderly people applying for Homes. Multi-disciplinary assessment seems essential.
- Some people want to move on from residential care and have the capacity to do so. It is important that those with hopes for change and progress are helped to find alternatives.

WHERE TO LEARN MORE

Some of the research about admission to Homes is succinctly reviewed in:

National Institute for Social Work(1988) *Residential Care for Elderly People: Using Research to Improve Practice,* London: NISW.

A more extended discussion, with a checklist of key points for managing admissions, can be found in:

Lawrence, S., Walker, A. and Willcocks, D. (1987) *She's Leaving Home,* Polytechnic of North London.

A detailed research report with many implications for practice is:

Neill, J. *et al.* (1988) *A Need for Care? Elderly Applicants for Local Authority Homes,* London: Avebury.

General discussion of principles and practice in admission and leaving care can be found in:

Brearley, P. *et al.* (1980) *Admission to Residential Care,* London: Tavistock Publications.
Brearley, P. *et al.* (1982) *Leaving Residential Care,* London: Tavistock Publications.

Chapter Six

'IF IT WERE YOUR MOTHER, OR BROTHER, OR FATHER . . .' : HELPING INDIVIDUALS

The basic principles of good practice have been established throughout the earlier discussions. This chapter considers the implications for individuals. Major considerations when elderly people arrive at the Home will be:

1 Listening to what the elderly person says, and understanding what she wants.
2 Enabling her to retain a sense of control over her own life and future plans.
3 Listening to what other 'customers' are saying. The family, friends, neighbours will have expectations and needs which must be taken into account. Field social workers, doctors, nurses, home helps, etc., will also have continuing interests and responsibilities which have to be included in planning.
4 Having clear plans and objectives, discussed and agreed with the elderly person.
5 Remembering the basic principles, and behaving respectfully, offering choice and treating people as individuals.

RECOGNIZING DIFFERENCES AND PRESERVING IDENTITY

People come to Homes in very different circumstances. The elderly person moving into a Home may have been considering coming for some time and have been waiting anxiously for the change. She may have come in as the result of an emergency and be bewildered, unsure or confused. The increasing use of residential Homes to provide short-stay care means that a growing proportion of people have had some experience of the Home – or a

Home – before coming in permanently. If the process has been well managed she will have met at least one member of staff and hopefully have visited the Home beforehand.

Whatever the process, the first few days and weeks will be a difficult and worrying time. It will help if staff can understand how it feels: we can all find memories of life experiences which help us understand what it is like – starting a new job, first days at school, etc. There are some very specific ways in which staff can help to reduce the stress and ease entry into the new situation: learning what is expected; physical appearance; and finding out who they are.

Learning what is expected

All Homes have a set of informal rules and behaviours, from favourite armchairs of established residents, to use of toilets, which television programme is watched in a particular lounge, etc. Some of the potential clashes with the habits of those who are already living in the Home can be offset by showing the newcomer to a 'safe corner' and making sure she understands what to do and where to go and what time to get meals, for instance. Introducing her to another resident who 'knows the ropes' and who can introduce her to others and to the usual ways of doing things, can be a simple way of getting over the first hurdles. It can also help to give the existing resident a feeling of purposefulness and value.

Physical appearance

A central element of self-esteem is feeling that the way you present yourself to the world is in your own control. Some people place much more store by how they look than others, but most would want to be well dressed and groomed and to look, in particular, *appropriately* dressed. By definition, those who come into Homes are usually at a time of reduced personal abilities and strengths. Many have been through a process of declining ability to look after themselves and may therefore have been unable to keep up the standards of personal cleanliness, hygiene and clothing that they would want. First impressions are important: it is important for helpers, whether family, home help, field social worker or residential worker, to put effort into helping the new resident prepare for the move, including giving guidance on personal clothing and cleanliness. Thereafter, residents need the facilities to buy and to keep their clothing neat and clean, with help with laundry and mending, if necessary (although many will be willing and able to do some, or all of this themselves). This certainly means clothes of their own – not the leavings of a previous resident.

Maintaining a good physical appearance is not just about clothing. Most Homes have a hairdresser visiting regularly and this can be a great boost to self-esteem. Some residents will prefer to go out to the hairdresser and should be helped to do so if necessary. Teeth are an important part of appearance and self-presentation and false teeth should be clean and well fitting. Provision of make-up and other personal toiletries is very important but is often inadequate because of limited income of individuals and failure of staff to see the need. Men should be able to shave or be shaved every day (unless they choose to grow a beard) and women too may need help with unwanted facial hair.

Although these may seem relatively minor issues, they can be of major importance in enabling people to present themselves as they wish to be. They are, therefore, fundamental aspects of an individualized approach.

Finding out who they are

A new resident will be bringing with her some 80 years or so of life experience. This is valuable from several points of view: it contributes to the life of the Home and the resources that the whole group has open to it and it also offers a basis for getting to know each person. There are at least three sorts of questions which it might be helpful to ask: Where is she from? What has she done? Who is she from?

In many Homes the majority of residents will have experiences of the nearby locality in common. Some may have been friends before, or even gone to school together. Others may have totally different life experiences to draw from, whether they be of Africa, the Punjab, or the English Midlands. All this helps staff to understand her and her needs and expectations and gives them a link to build on with other members of the resident group.

We all try to identify ourselves by the kinds of roles we play: bus driver, care assistant, mother, daughter, home help, etc. We use this to reinforce our understanding of who we are and how we fit into the world and to explain these things to other people. People are more than the sum of the roles that they perform in society, but roles are nevertheless very important to us in 'locating' ourselves amongst others. Elderly people tend to lose roles as they grow older through retirement, bereavement, and other losses. Coming into a Home they lose other important roles: householder, tenant, shopper, neighbour. Exploring with each resident the roles and tasks she has successfully carried out in the past can be a way of building self-esteem. There is further discussion of the value of reminiscence later in the book. Getting a picture of past history helps also to build up respect and understanding. To know that Mrs Edwards was a police officer, or that Mrs French raised eight children after her husband's death is bound to help staff to relate to that woman's needs and behaviour in a more understanding way.

The question 'Who is she from?' is rather more complex. It concerns family background and relationships. It is common when new residents arrive for other residents to seek common acquaintances ('Who do you know?') as a way of making contact. More broadly, it is important to know who is or has been important to residents both in their past life and in the present. The influence of a long-dead mother, father or husband can continue to have major impact on elderly people that can be just as important as that of a daughter who visits regularly, or another who never comes at all. If staff are to understand and help they need some of this background.

There was discussion in Chapter 2 of what has become known as the biographical approach to understanding ageing: a way of understanding people through their life history. Staff of Homes can use a similar approach in getting to know individual residents. It is common practice in child care for workers to help children find and record the continuity of their life in care by building up a scrapbook or other 'life-story book' about their own history. A similar approach is helpful in residential care for elderly people.

This is not necessarily to suggest that all residents should be helped to create a personal life-history book. For some this may be appropriate and many will, of course, have this in the form of photograph albums and other 'paper memories'. Rather, it is a suggestion that residential workers should actively set out to learn from residents about what is important to them.

One helpful way to do this is to begin with the life story: not all at once but at the right pace for each person. This is a way to begin a relationship, to find helpful ways of improving their lives and to provide information to help other staff see each resident in the light of all they have been and have achieved in the past – not just as one more frail, elderly person.

MAKING CONTACT: COMMUNICATION

In order to help with some of these things and to make first contacts with residents, staff need to have skills in communicating. For the great majority of people the fact that they are chronologically older is not an important factor in the way they communicate. Some, however, do find that in later life they experience specific communication problems and some understanding of what creates or increases these is essential.

Sensory loss

People are likely to experience deterioration in sensory abilities as they age. Of all the sensory problems, hearing impairment is likely to be the most devastating to the process of communication. There have, in fact, been relatively few studies of the incidence of deafness and there is some uncertainty about its incidence among the very elderly, but it seems likely that about one-third of older people in the general community have some degree of hearing impairment. The majority of hard-of-hearing people are elderly. It has been estimated that 70 per cent of people over the age of 70 have a significant hearing loss. This rises to 84 per cent at 85 years and over (Social Services Inspectorate 1988). Elderly people in hospitals and other institutional settings have an even greater chance of experiencing moderate or severe hearing loss.

The deafness which tends to accompany old age, presbyacusis, has two main characteristics: there is a progressive deterioration with age of the ability to hear high frequencies, and there is a greater sensitivity to loud noises. Two problems are common. Since consonants tend to be high pitched and vowel sounds of lower pitch, older people with hearing loss often receive only unintelligible vowel sounds. Second, there is often a difficulty in separating out different sounds: the 'cocktail party effect' in which all sounds are received in the same way and speech cannot be selected from background noise. One 88-year-old lady described how this affected her when using her hearing-aid, which tends to emphasize this difficulty:

> Two friends came to visit me. I had not expected them, and I had perhaps put my hearing aid up rather louder for some reason or another (perhaps I was listening to the radio, and doing something else). I came into the sitting room with my friends and talked to them – and found I was hearing the clock on the mantelpiece very distinctly. I said to my friends, 'Excuse me, I can hear the clock far too distinctly. I must adjust my hearing aid' and they both said, 'We did not hear it at all'. Now, they did not hear it, not because their hearing was defective, but because their hearing was too good. In other words, their ears were accommodating themselves to extraneous sounds and shutting them out, and they were only listening to the conversation.
>
> (Goodrich 1976)

Discomfort, associated with wax in the ears or with 'recruitment' (the fact that loud sounds can be painful), or with tinnitus (the various whistling or hissing noises sometimes associated with deafness), is also an important feature. When communicating with an older person with hearing impairment it is important to speak clearly and distinctly, but not loudly, and to face the older person to facilitate lip-reading. Keep extraneous noises to a minimum: a radio or television, for instance, can be a block to reception of speech. Avoid smoking or covering the mouth in any way and emphasize points by gesture or expression. If the elderly person is not receiving important information this can be written down or questions or comments rephrased. It is important not to assume that a message has been understood and it may be useful to ask the resident to repeat important information to ensure it has been received.

Particularly important are practical aids to communication. If a hearing-aid is available this should be kept in good repair and used; similarly, if spectacles are available then they should be worn.

An induction loop system is particularly useful in Homes. Dentures should also be remembered: speech can be improved and embarrassment reduced if the older person has her teeth in.

Impairment of vision is also commonly associated with ageing. Some sight changes appear to happen to everyone. Over the age of about 45, most people experience some degree of long-sightedness, although almost perfect sight may continue throughout life. The processes of age-related change are usually complex: changes in the retina, fading of the iris, thickening of the cornea and changes in the nervous system may all contribute. Changes are also complicated by variations in alertness and attention which affect perceptual ability. Visual disability in elderly people is commonly caused by glaucoma, cataract or macular disease, but these may cause varying and fluctuating effects. There may be considerable changes in visual difficulties throughout the day, and changes in ability to see are not just, as is often assumed, about willingness to see ('She can see when she really wants to . . .').

The importance of blindness to communication difficulties is obvious and it is particularly important among those who experience a degree of both hearing and vision impairment. A blind person is unable to recognize people and therefore the initiative in beginning contact usually rests on others. It is important, therefore, for a worker to announce her presence and purpose clearly at the beginning of contact and to inform the older person if they are joined by someone else. The use of other senses must be maximized: clear and distinct speech, and the tone of voice contribute to conveying a message. Lighting is also important: avoid sitting against the light or in a glaring light. Good lighting and use of colours, for instance, is necessary to enable people to make best use of the sight that is left.

Difficulties in use or understanding of language may also occur since ageing people are particularly susceptible to neurological degeneration and disease. There may be a difficulty in forming words and speech or the problem may be in understanding language. The loss of the power to actually understand or make sense of language is likely to be a particularly frightening and disturbing experience for the individual: 'Suddenly he lives in a world of scrambled communication' (McCall 1979). A person with speech difficulties will speak better if he is able to initiate the conversation in a familiar and comfortable environment. Visual cues and gestures, shorter, clearly articulated words and as many visual, non-spoken cues as possible will help in getting the meaning across. There will be people in Homes whose first language is not English. There should be opportunities for them to speak to people who share their language; where there are larger minority groups it is important to employ staff from the same group to enable a proper understanding of their language and other cultural needs.

Other aspects of health or illness are likely to contribute to communication difficulties. Discomfort arising from pain or tiredness will influence how people talk. Limitations of mobility and balance also have effects. An overall strategy for communication should recognize the impact of these factors and look for common-sense solutions. If someone is tired then try again some other time; if she has difficulties in movement on one side of her body, then don't sit on that side, etc.

Changes in mood or emotional expression may also be affected by physical disease or deterioration. The fact that someone bursts into tears does not necessarily mean that she is deeply distressed, and it is therefore necessary to look carefully at the relationships between context, attitudes, responses, and expressions to understand the true meaning. Some behaviour is described as confused: this term may be used to describe a number of features, including difficulties in remembering, disturbance in general orientation, and agitation. Such behaviour may be symptomatic of dementia, or of physical illness, or it may be a consequence of depression; sometimes it is the result of sudden change. Whatever the cause it is important to give the older person *time* to consider and understand what is to be communicated.

It should never be assumed that an older person cannot understand: events have some meaning even to the person with advanced brain failure. At one end of the scale, this may mean reminding a forgetful resident that it is time for her favourite television programme; at the other end, it may mean giving a severely demented older person time to accustom herself to the idea of getting out of bed rather than simply pulling back the bedclothes and helping her up immediately. This is discussed in more detail later.

Recognizing the age-gap

Older people and their carers, themselves often in late middle age or older, may perceive some things differently because of their different life experiences. At its simplest this may lead to them expressing a preference for an older worker. One writer reports the case of a depressed woman of 58 caring for her 88-year-old mother. Her first meeting with a social worker was short and she regarded the age and sex of the social worker as off-putting, although Rees suggests that ultimately such a reaction was unimportant: 'I thought he was very young for the job and didn't actually think he'd get anything done. I'm being perfectly honest, he seemed a bit wary of approaching my mother. He says he's going to do something. I'm surprised' (Rees 1978: 79).

A different aspect of the age-gap between older people at risk and professional workers is the time factor. It was suggested earlier in the book that it seems reasonable to speculate that an hour in the life of a lonely, isolated person is likely to be experienced very differently by that person than that hour is experienced in the life of a busy visitor, even though they may spend the same hour together. Similarly, ten minutes of the time of a head of Home is likely to have much more significance to the resident with whom she spends the time. Although there is little clear evidence that this is a substantial feature of communication it must be an element to be taken into account when estimating the meaning of experiences.

Time is also understood historically, and the fact that older people have lived through different experiences to those of younger people has some implications. Gray, for example, suggests that words may have different meanings since their usage has changed over recent years. She suggests that phrases such as 'he was hurt in an accident', rather than 'injured', or 'I see what you mean', rather than 'perceive', are preferable for this reason. Other examples relate to the use of words common among professionals – such as 'discharge', 'admission', 'part III', 'accommodation' – which may be unfamiliar to the older person and should therefore be avoided. Similarly, local expressions or sayings may be familiar to some but not others (Gray and Isaacs 1979).

A similar point relates to the general presentation and manners of the worker. Older people may be less accustomed to the casual approach or forms of dress used by many workers. The potential meanings of such aspects should always be borne in mind.

Improving communication

The most important point of all is to begin with the elderly person and her perception of the situation. For the worker, some simple prescriptions for practical communication can be listed. McCall gives a very useful checklist for talking to someone with hearing loss. She suggests the following as important: to give warning; avoid startling; gain attention before speaking; light should not be focused on your face; aim for quiet circumstances; make the subject known at the beginning of a conversation; speak in sentences, not one word at a time, at a reasonable speed; if you are not understood, change the sentence round; never shout; and, above all, recognize that privacy matters and that communication should be improved by tactful and unobtrusive means (McCall 1979).

More generally, it is essential to move at the resident's pace. Communication may need to be slower and more precise for the elderly person. The deterioration of sensory and perceptual capacities among elderly people means that non-verbal cues take on greater importance. Silence is not uncommon and patience is necessary. Sometimes physical touch is one way of contributing to reassurance or trust. Although there are social and sexual taboos involved in touch between adults, if it is sensitively used, touch can help. The following example, although drawn from field social work, is an illustration of how this can help:

Mrs Green had been admitted to hospital following an overdose taken as a result of the mounting pressure of caring for her husband, several years older than herself and seriously ill. After her return home he was admitted to hospital and died shortly afterwards. She neither visited him in hospital nor attended his funeral.

Two years after his death she requested help from the Social Services Department with finances and the social worker noted that the crisis arose two days after the anniversary of the husband's death. During her early contacts with Mrs Green the social worker focused mainly on the practical issues – payment of a gas bill, repairs of the fire, etc.

She soon became aware of oblique references to guilt, anxiety and grief in Mrs Green's conversation. As the worker expressed it: 'I had the overwhelming feeling that on one level she was warning me off the subject, but on another she desperately wanted to talk about it'.

After a number of visits which included planning a trip to the crematorium where her husband had been cremated and developing discussion of her feelings about her husband, the worker noted at the end of one visit: 'Mrs Green had also mentioned a suitcase which had remained unopened since Mr Green's death and also a wedding photograph, both of which evoked the same response of anxiety and fear in her ... After this visit, Mrs Green gave me a very warm hug and I felt that this was her way of expressing relief that she would be allowed to examine her worst fears'.

Soon afterwards she added: 'Through these painful experiences we seemed to reach a point of togetherness and the hug became our weekly farewell. I didn't feel it was indicative of too much dependence on the relationship as it always felt spontaneous and right and the communication expressed could not be equally conveyed in words.'

Communication: improving the environment

Three particular elements can be emphasized:

1 Improving the 'interpersonal environment' for communication. This involves helping to make people available to the older person for communication and enabling those people to contribute to overcoming the barriers to effective communication by support, and by teaching skills of communication. Some of the commonest barriers may not even be recognized. In one small study of deafness, for instance, in residential Homes for elderly people, it was found that over 27 per cent of those who were severely impaired were not identified as such by staff of the Homes. Impairment was found to be more likely to be recognized when residents wore a hearing-aid, admitted to the handicap, and were known to the member of staff for a longer time. Older staff were more successful in identifying impaired residents, and men were less likely to be

recognized as impaired than women (Martin and Peckford 1978). The fact that such a large minority of people with hearing impairment are not identified must be a matter of considerable concern and points to a need for training in this aspect of work in particular.

2 Providing practical aids to overcome sensory loss and encouragement in using them.

3 Improving the overall environment. The organization of Homes to reduce danger to people with poor sight – no loose carpets, good lighting, ensuring everything returns to an accustomed place, etc. – and overcoming problems of acoustic design of residential Homes, providing equipment to help with hearing difficulties and improve the use of television, etc., are important. At least as important is to improve understanding of the problems of communication for older people.

To summarize, it is necessary to begin by engaging the older person. It is not enough to work just with the *ability* to communicate: *motivation* to communicate is probably as important to many. Elderly people in Homes are likely to be frail, with sensory loss, and their skills of communication may have deteriorated through disuse, as may their will to be involved with others. They may no longer want to make the effort. If older people *want* to be involved with others they are, of course, more likely to maintain and practise their communication skills.

PERSONAL CARE: REACHING AN AGREEMENT

People enter residential care because they are in need of help with personal care tasks which they cannot manage themselves. Few people now go into Homes in either the public or private sectors unless they need quite substantial help with personal care. A first stage in settling in should therefore be to bring together the previous assessment and objectives set before admission with the growing understanding of the residential staff in order to plan for the best way to provide care. It is most appropriate to think of this as a 'Care Agreement' to be reached between the Home and the resident. This has sometimes been called a 'Care Plan'.

There will be several elements to the Care Agreement:

1 What the resident has been led to expect from previous discussions and from any published brochure about the Home which will have described some of the minimum standards she can expect.
2 Any contract or terms and conditions of residence agreed at the point of admission. In the Local Authority Home this will be at the very least a statement of how much the weekly charge will be. It may include a number of other elements in the private sector. *Home Life*, for instance, proposes that 'all residents, and where necessary their spouses as well, should be given in writing a clear statement of the terms under which the accommodation is offered' (Centre for Policy on Ageing 1984: p62). This would include such things as a statement on what the resident will be expected to provide for herself, circumstances in which she might be asked to leave, procedures for making complaints, services covered by fees, and procedures for increasing fees, etc.
3 A process of discussing and learning about each other by staff and residents during the first few weeks.

At the end of a period of around six weeks (between four and eight weeks, depending on circumstances) a review should be held in which all parties should take part and should be able to contribute to planning for the future. A major part of this plan should be an agreement on the type of care to be provided and how it is to be given. This agreement should be reviewed periodically but should be flexible enough to be developed informally as necessary.

Personal and physical care

There are certain things that everyone needs to be able to do to live a reasonably ordinary life. These include eating, sleeping, moving around, being comfortable, warm and reasonably safe. Some people are unable to perform the tasks that surround these activities: feeding, dressing, washing, going to the toilet, etc. These are usually known as self-care tasks and are concerned with the most intimate aspects of life which most people, for most of their lives, do themselves. Elderly people in Homes need help from other people with some or most self-care tasks, because of physical or mental frailty, or disability.

The concepts of personal care, health, well-being and illness are closely bound up together. Many people may need help with some self-care tasks such as putting on stockings, tying shoelaces, getting in and out of the bath or handling cutlery. This is not the same as being ill and needing treatment from a doctor. Being old is not an illness. Nevertheless, the boundaries of nursing care and personal care can be blurred in residential Homes. The Registered Homes Act (1984) enables private and voluntary homes to seek to be registered as both a Residential Care Home and a Nursing Home and to provide both 'personal care and board' and nursing care. Local Authority Homes often provide care for people with, for example, pressure sores, or needing daily injections, who are receiving substantial help from Community Nursing Services.

It is important to be clear about where the boundaries are. On the one hand residential workers should not treat people as 'patients' when they are providing personal care help. On the other hand, they should not obstruct residents' proper medical care because of over-rejection of the 'medical model' of care. Residents should receive sensitive and tactful help with intimate personal care tasks but should also have access to nursing and health care when illness or other treatable conditions warrant it: just as someone in their own home would receive care.

It is not the purpose of this book to give detailed guidance on how to provide personal care help. There are other sources of clear guidance. There are, however, some central aspects of daily living which are of particular importance and which will be discussed to illustrate some issues about attitudes and approaches.

Being able to move around

When someone lives in her own home there will be a good deal of physical activity throughout the day, however frail she might be. Moving to toilet or commode, making a sandwich, answering the door, washing and dressing all provide regular, routine exercise. In a residential Home there are people to do many of these tasks for residents. The hotel element of service can detract from the quality of opportunity to exercise in a myriad of little ways. If the only exercise is dressing, walking to a lounge, to the toilet, to the dining-room, back to the lounge and then to bed, then physical abilities are likely to deteriorate.

Exercise is essential and natural opportunities to take exercise should be built in to the daily life of the Home. These should be based on things people want to do. Motivation is most important.

The furnishings and the environment make an important contribution. Chairs, for instance can be a dilemma: efforts to provide a domestic appearance to lounges may lead to low-level armchairs which are virtually impossible to get out of without help. There are many well-designed chairs which are comfortable, enable people to stand up more easily, yet look good. Different places to sit within the Home, with interesting views of the outside or different activities, will encourage people to move around during the day. Corridors should not be too long or 'staging-posts' may be needed so people can take a rest on very long stretches. Floors should be clean, dry and safe. Rugs, loose carpets, or wet vinyl are extremely dangerous.

Equipment to help people should be a basic consideration. Walking sticks, frames and other aids should be appropriate to the individual, who should be given training in how to use them properly. At the most basic, footwear should enable, not hinder, mobility. Loose house slippers may be comfortable for sitting but increase difficulty walking and reduce confidence.

People will not walk comfortably if their feet hurt. Good chiropody is essential to mobility for many. Where necessary, staff should help residents to ensure that feet are in good condition and get professional help where appropriate.

The basics of providing the best possible mobility, then, are:

- confidence and motivation;
- a safe and suitable environment;
- proper exercise and personal and health care for feet etc;
- appropriate equipment and furnishings.

Eating well

The main periods of activity for most people in most Homes are around mealtimes. Meals are a social event and should be treated as such: they should not be rushed for staff convenience but should be a leisurely and relaxed opportunity for people to eat with friends. The implications of this for presentation of meals are obvious: there should be attractive tables, laid in a homely manner. Putting out food on each plate at a serving hatch and plonking the plate in front of residents is unacceptable. Tureens, teapots and milk jugs enable people to help each other and themselves to what they want. If this leads to disputes in some cases, that is not a reason to return to institutionalized ready-plated food but points to a need for discussion and perhaps reorganizing seating or providing more food to some tables.

Real choice of food means having at least two types available for people to pick from. It is not enough to say 'They could have something else if they asked for it': real choice means telling and preferably showing people what is actually available to them.

Food should be varied, nutritious and clean. Choice can be offered in various ways: by residents' involvement in menu-planning, by having more than one meal available, by offering a choice in advance and cooking to individual orders, or by using a microwave and frozen food for snack meals etc. People should be able to eat at a different time from the majority in some circum-stances. Cooks may only be employed from 8.30a.m. to 4.30p.m. but systems can easily be devised to provide an evening meal if a resident goes shopping with her daughter. There should also be enough flexibility for residents to have a fish and chip supper from time to time, or a pub meal occasionally. Food should reflect the personal and cultural preferences of residents. This needs to take account of local patterns of eating and recipes and also the special dietary needs of members of black and ethnic minority groups. Staff should be trained to understand and respond to these needs.

Some residents need help with feeding. The first question should be whether equipment such as specialist cutlery would enable them to manage alone. If they do need someone to help, this should be done sensitively and unobtrusively. Staff should not be feeding several people at once and serving meals at the same time. If staff time is short and demand high, then consider other solutions. Can rotas be varied? Does the meal need to be over so quickly? Could volunteers help with feeding? Can some residents eat separately or at another time?

The basics of providing food, then, include:

- attractive, varied, nutritious, clean food;
- real choice of actual alternatives for residents;
- a flexible approach to people who need help;
- making meals a social occasion for residents, with food served in a homelike manner.

Dressing, bathing and toilet

Some of the most intimate kinds of help surround the need for assistance with bodily functions. The right to privacy must begin at this basic level: ensuring that people receive help which intrudes as little as possible on privacy. This means providing private places to dress and wash and involving no more people than absolutely necessary in providing the help.

The basic practicalities must be in place first. Toilet doors should be screened from main living areas. They should be large enough for people in wheelchairs to get in and shut the door behind them and designed to enable them to transfer across independently if possible. Doors should be lockable. Equipment should be appropriate and up-to-date. Various designs of special baths are available: both staff and residents vary widely in their attitudes to these: sometimes ordinary 'island' baths are preferred because they involve personal contact between staff and residents. Sometimes hoists or special baths are preferred for the opposite reason. The important point is that there should be choice for the residents.

Staff often feel a responsibility to make sure that everyone takes a bath regularly. This leads to 'bath books', weight charts and other institutionalized practices. The obligation is to provide appropriate apparatus for residents to maintain personal hygiene as they wish: if they want to do this by a strip-wash in their own room, that must be for them to decide. There may be some who are too confused to decide for themselves and who need tactful encouragement. Occasionally, some may need encouragement to improve their hygiene for the sake of other residents but this will be very exceptional. It is of fundamental importance that elderly people retain control of what is done to their bodies – even if they need help in doing it.

Doing things for residents is often quite simple. It is easy to button up a blouse, fasten a skirt. It may take much longer to stand back and encourage or guide that person to do it for themselves. But often the latter is the best course of action. If skills are not used, they deteriorate; if muscles are not exercised, they atrophy. There will always be a fine balance between doing things for people and doing things with them. Care staff will need to discuss amongst themselves and agree with residents the most appropriate way of helping. The worst reaction is probably to refuse to help and walk away, leaving someone to struggle 'for their own good': that is the route to frustration, anger or despair. Encouraging residents to do things for themselves means looking for easier strategies, making sure clothing is comfortable and easy to manage, finding equipment to help them put on stockings or shoes, etc., and, above all, being alongside them whilst they cope.

Personal care: a summary

These examples of personal care involvement – mobility, food and personal toilet and dressing – have begun to illustrate the important principles of approach which can be applied to other kinds of care help:

1 Do things differently if people's needs are different: don't assume everyone needs help with bathing; don't expect everyone to be grateful; allow people to have different abilities and attitudes to being dependent.
2 Remember elderly people can change from day to day and throughout the day. Sometimes people would like to lie in bed, or a bit of help with their buttons: it helps to keep up the longer-term struggle if there is an occasional luxury.
3 Make sure the environment is as good as it can be: avoid traps like rugs and loose carpets and provide colour variation to help people find their way around.
4 Get equipment to help people do it for themselves wherever possible – and get good advice on what is available. Make sure residents are taught how to use it and given support and encouragement if they are unsure. A lot of equipment is unused through lack of training and confidence.
5 Be flexible: let people lead lives that are different from the majority if they wish. If a resident wants to go to bed after midnight make arrangements for help to be available: don't make her fit around shifts for staff convenience.
6 Give real choice: don't wait for people to ask. Offer options and show residents what is available if possible. There is no choice if they do not know what is available.
7 Above all, be tactful, sensitive and respectful – especially of personal privacy: screen washbasins in double rooms, screen

commodes and empty pans discreetly, assume that no one wants an audience when they are having a bath.

ILL HEALTH AND ILLNESS

These principles of good care apply also to ways of approaching health care and illness. It would not be appropriate to review here the range of health problems and illnesses that affect elderly people in Homes. Some general aspects of making health care arrangements and approaching resident care can, however, be illustrated.

Amongst a group of frail, very elderly people living together it is likely that some illness or disease will be present most of the time. In large groups illnesses may commonly be passed around by infection. The residential worker must therefore be alert to recognizing physical changes and must routinely observe residents. A resident's appearance may show changes in a range of ways, such as skin colour and texture, weight change and mood. There may be changes in energy, interest and intellectual ability which may indicate some underlying problem. A general awareness of each resident on a day-to-day basis is essential, as well as a readiness to recognize and respond to specific complaints or symptoms.

A particular issue for many residents is maintaining continence. Probably around a quarter of residents in most Homes are reported to be often incontinent, especially of urine, and a similar proportion experience occasional incontinence. This is distressing and uncomfortable for the resident and those around her. The issues surrounding the management of continence provide a helpful illustration of responding to health care issues more generally. Mandelstam (1985) has written helpfully about incontinence. She points out the importance of proper assessment of the cause of incontinence. She suggests an eight-point list for the physiotherapist, within the multi-disciplinary team in which the nurse is responsible for initial assessment, toilet regimes and the use of equipment. In the residential Home, staff will need to involve community nurses and GP in assessment but can achieve a great deal by taking account of the following points, based loosely on Mandelstam's approach.

1 The need to monitor the pattern of micturition, to chart it and see what the chart shows (but please keep charts in a

private place!). Decisions can then be made about whether the usual toileting arrangements meet the resident's needs and whether a different toilet regime would help.

2 If residents have difficulty in communicating because, for instance, of aphasia, then ways of signalling a need by perhaps a bell or card saying 'Toilet, please' should be explored. Do experiment.

3 If there are problems of motor or sensory disturbance following, for example, a stroke, then the actual mechanics of using a lavatory may need to be relearned.

4 Access to the toilet should be quick and simple: can it be improved?

5 Consider the use of a commode, of the right height to transfer from a bed or chair.

6 Ensure privacy: this is of fundamental importance.

7 Clothes should be easy to manage: can they be removed as quickly as necessary?

8 If the resident cannot be helped to remain continent following assessment, then there should be further assessment of the best kind of equipment to assist.

The first step must be assessment: if the cause can be identified appropriate treatment may remove the problem. If not it can be managed to provide major improvements.

Similar principles apply to other health issues. Elderly residents are often unable to perform physical movements which are essential to carrying out basic daily tasks. If these are viewed as performance problems there are broadly two essential lines of approach. First, assess the underlying cause and, if necessary, seek medical help to do this properly. Similarly, assess ways in which the performance can be improved and problems managed: this may be done in three main ways:

1 By therapy: occupational therapists, physiotherapists, speech therapists, etc., can make an enormous difference to the abilities of elderly people to perform tasks and cope with the environment. Although paramedical services are often in short supply in the community every effort should be made to provide their help to residents in Homes.

2 By providing equipment to make the task easier.

3 By changing the environment. 'Don't raise the bridge, lower the road': a little creative thinking can often reduce the lack of 'fit' between the resident and her environment.

If medical help is needed it should be remembered that it is the resident and doctor who need to communicate. Some residents will want to contact the surgery direct or to visit the doctor at the surgery. Many will ask staff to make an appointment for them. When the doctor visits he should be able to see the resident alone or in the residents own room, unless the resident asks for staff to be present.

Managing medication for residents is a complex matter. If residents want to keep their own medicines they should not be prevented from doing so, but should be able to keep them in a secure, locked place. If staff keep medicines they should keep a full record of what is received, when it is administered to each resident, and when any is disposed of. The advice of a pharmacist can be invaluable in finding ways of encouraging independence where possible but ensuring secure administration of drugs as necessary.

Treatment and medication should be regularly reviewed. Often, residential staff need to prompt review by doctors of medication. They should be alert to possible side effects of drugs and be prepared to question treatment on behalf of residents if they feel it necessary.

EMOTIONAL AND RELATIONSHIP NEEDS

Providing for the personal and physical care needs of residents is not just about a physical exchange but inevitably leads to the growth of close relationships. In some ways, the dependence which grows between staff and residents is similar to that between parent and child. The closer the relationship becomes, the more confused people may become about which role they are actually playing: the discrepancy between ages of carer and cared-for contributes to this.

Sometimes staff may begin to feel they are filling the role of daughter, but some elderly people may begin to regress in their behaviour and treat staff almost like a parent. It is helpful to think about how relationships develop and can be used to help residents in terms of at least four different sorts of dimensions of need. First, there are needs and wants which are mainly focused on the self. Second, there are needs which are focused outwards, on the external world. Third, needs arise from pressures in the present, here and now. Fourth, needs also arise from experiences in the past. In order to understand relationships each of these dimensions should be taken into account.

Some elements of this will be discussed further in relation to the experience of living in a group. As far as individuals are concerned, each resident will have needs for affection and satisfying personal relationships, just as people of any age need love and friendship. Staff will need to demonstrate their feeling that all residents are valued for their individual worth and that they are accepted as whole people, including their less pleasant and even unsociable habits. Some residents may indulge in these as a way of testing staff's real attitudes. This may be seen after admission when they need recovery time to build up strengths, but it may also be seen later as relationships become very close, and inappropriate behaviour may develop as dependency increases either because of increased mental infirmity or because of a testing of relationships.

It will be necessary to set some limits: to find the balanced use of authority to check exaggerated behaviour and to promote group and individual satisfactions. Residents should be treated with consistency and respect and workers may need to explore with residents their feelings about the limitations being placed on them.

Reference was made earlier to Erikson's (1964) concept of ego-development and the life-cycle. This offers a helpful way of thinking about the meaning to elderly people of past and present. Erikson proposes that there are eight major stages to be negotiated in the process of personal development through life. The final stage involves achieving an integrated state of mind through the resolution of a conflict between ego-integrity and despair. It means, in Erikson's terms, accepting one's one and only life-cycle as something that had to be and that, by necessity, permitted of no substitution. Despair represents the feeling that life is too short to make up the deficits in past life: it involves, in other words, the fear of death.

There are difficulties in following Erikson's approach too literally, although it is an approach that is well worth detailed study. The simple proposition that elderly people need to be able to look back on life and see a purpose and meaning is of central importance. The use of reminiscence in counselling is one way to help residents to understand how they come to be where they are, to review past success and achievements and to accept what they have not been able to achieve. For many, the real physical and material limitations and deprivation of opportunities will contribute to feelings of unhappiness and despair. This can be offset by a balanced discussion of achievements and by opportunities to do valued and useful things in the present. Reminiscence is discussed further in the following chapter.

The issue of dying and bereavement will be developed to illustrate some of the ways of helping in relation to feelings, attitudes and emotions.

Dealing with death and dying is a central part of residential care. Most residents know that they are there until they die and Homes have sometimes been called 'anterooms to death'. Death and dying are, therefore, a common part of life in residential care and different establishments find different ways of dealing with it. The awareness of death can actually give an intensity and meaning to the life that is left.

Most elderly residents will feel a need to talk about death at some time and to review their feelings about the approach of death. Some will say that they are ready for death, that they feel they have lived a good and useful life and are 'ready to go'. 'I wish he'd come and take me' is a common comment, and sometimes this may seem a realistic and calm acceptance. However, a substantial number of people in Homes are depressed, and apparent disinterest in life may be related to that depression. An apathetic acceptance of impending death should ring warning bells: treatment for depression may lead to a renewed interest in life opportunities. The skill for the residential worker is in knowing how to distinguish between realistic acceptance which can be encouraged by individual and group discussion (when the residents make this possible) and depression.

The decision about whether or not a person who is in the terminal stage of illness should stay in the Home or go to hospital is often difficult. A residential Home may not be equipped for the nursing tasks needed and staff may feel anxious or fear accusations from relatives that all had not been done that should have been done. Discussions of what to do should be held with doctor, community nurse, family and the resident if possible.

If the resident is dying in the Home she should continue to be treated as a whole person and not as a dying body. Anxiety and distress in the dying person tend to be associated with physical distress or pain (or fear of pain). Successful treatment of physical distress will ease the emotional distress. Many people who are dying appreciate the opportunity to discuss their feelings with a sympathetic listener. Residential staff can help to create a climate in which the resident feels free to discuss her feelings about impending death. Discussion may need to include plans for surviving family or friends. A clear understanding about what will happen when she is dead, that the will is in order, the burial or cremation arrangements agreed, will give relief to both resident and relatives.

Much depends, of course, on whether death can be anticipated or whether it comes quickly. Some people anticipate death calmly, and as long as they do not expect pain, they approach dying quite gently. A quiet, calm death is easier for those who are around the resident, but it is not necessarily the only, 'good' way to die. Some people face death with anger and resistance: this should not be seen as a 'bad' way to die. The important thing for most people is that someone stays alongside them. Helping the dying resident will require an ability to be aware of her feelings about death and separate those from the worker's own fears. It is no help to say, 'I know how you feel. If I were you I would be frightened too.' It may be helpful to say, 'I think I know how you feel but I care enough to stay and help you with your fears.'

It is important also to get the practicalities of care right. Follow the medical guidance, keep people clean and comfortable, make sure the relatives are involved and kept informed, follow agreed routines after death, paying particular attention to religious and cultural preferences. Decide with other residents how to behave after the death. They will want to know what has happened and if the undertaker rushes the body out of the back door at 6 a.m. it may be a long time before most residents realize what has happened. Agree with them about what to do about the funeral, the flowers and the family. Some may want to attend the funeral and give flowers, etc. Some may feel that funeral flowers in the

Home are a morbid reminder that they do not want; others may find them a pleasant reminder of a loved friend and a help with coming to terms with loss. The principle to follow is not to make assumptions: talk to the residents about what they want to do.

Death is, of course, distressing for both staff and residents. Workers who have been closely involved in caring for a dying person and in dealing with death naturally feel upset: distress is inevitable and should be openly recognized and discussed. There is a temptation, when working with a group of people who are likely to die, to try to keep feelings at arm's length. This may be quite dangerous as a way of coping: a better strategy is likely to be to share feelings in an open and matter-of-fact way with colleagues. Senior staff should help to talk it through with staff groups and individuals as necessary.

There is general consensus that grief follows a typical course. Most people agree that normal grief is composed of different stages, although precise categorizations differ and often there is a cluster of symptoms by which we recognize grief in a general sense. In the usual course of events the bereaved person (or group of people) will pass through stages of denial, anger, depression and anguish as she continues to do the work of mourning and begins to cope with memories of the dead person. These patterns fluctuate. Some of the feelings will recur for years afterwards and staff should be alert to the importance of anniversaries of death, birthdays of a dead husband or wife, etc. These are times of particular pain of recurring grief.

The example of death and dying illustrates the ways in which residential workers may need to be able to help people cope with feelings from the past as well as current feelings and to relate these to the resident's needs both individually and within the group and the wider world of the Home.

Other emotional needs arising from intimate, trusting relationships and the need for respect and an individual response can be similarly understood. Issues arise, for example, from family and other community links, from the need for sexual relationships and expression, for religious activity and opportunity, etc. Although they cannot be discussed in detail here they should be approached on a similar basis:

• take account of past experiences as well as present needs;

- focus on the individual as well as the 'individual-in- the-group';
- get the practicalities of care right;
- deal respectfully with what each person wishes and needs;
- don't forget the needs of the larger group of residents.

CONTROL AND POWER

One final thing to think about when providing personal care help is the balance of power. It has several times been indicated earlier that a feeling of control is important to whether residents feel at ease with themselves and their life. In particular, if they feel that coming into the Home was their own choice and under their control and if they are able to control their immediate environment in the Home, they are more likely to feel satisfied.

It seems reasonable to assume that being in charge of their own lives, both their general destiny and the day-to-day details, will be important. Yet frail, elderly people are often very dependent on others for the most basic of things. If we are to improve their lives we must think, therefore, about how to give a reality of control or at the very least a feeling of being in control. There is an important role for independent advocates to be considered here.

One example of how control is exercised is the way in which money is managed. In many Homes, whether in the public or private sector, it is common for control of money to pass from resident to family or the Home manager on admission. This may be administratively efficient. It also 'removes the worry' from the residents, some of whom may feel quite happy about it. It does however, remove an important area of control. Receiving a small amount of personal allowance – or 'pocket money', as it is often (rather demeaningly) called – gives little feeling of control. Often the allowance is given out to suit the convenience of staff, and some may be retained where residents are judged unable to manage it themselves. Residential staff should think of ways in which greater control of their own money can be retained by residents. One way is to offer more opportunity to spend it as they wish: to help them get to shops to buy what they want. Again, the independent advocate can make an important contribution.

This is a complex area of practice. Residential workers should be guided by the principle that they are there to enable residents to do what they cannot do for themselves and to achieve what they want for themselves. Start from that perspective and some of the greater oppressions that can easily happen in Homes may be avoided. There are some complicating factors, especially the need to balance the rights of different residents in the same group and the need to find the balance between protection and safety. These are explored in more detail in the next chapter.

HELPING INDIVIDUALS: SUMMARY OF KEY POINTS

This chapter has considered the individual needs of elderly residents and some of the principles of practice to be borne in mind in providing personal, health and emotional care:

- It is essential to recognize the differences between people (including cultural and ethnic differences) and find ways of responding to each resident differently. One useful way of doing so is by exploring, with her, her life story. This helps staff to see what she brings with her to the Home.
- In order to make links with people on an individual basis, residential workers need to be able to communicate with elderly people. Communication is made more complicated because of the hearing, sight, and other sensory losses of elderly people. The key elements in good communication are people to talk to, practical equipment and a suitable physical environment in which lighting, colours, etc., enhance the remaining abilities.
- It is necessary to reach an agreement about care with the resident based on an assessment and shared understanding of her needs. This agreement should be renewed regularly and be flexible enough to change as necessary.
- Personal care help should be given on the basis of individual need which may change daily. The environment should be as good as possible in providing scope for residents to do as much as they can for themselves. Equipment to enhance self-care abilities should be provided. Above all help should be tactful, respectful and sensitively given.
- If people are ill, medical assessment should be sought. The input of paramedical professionals should be sought and their advice should be taken to improve the health and well-being of residents.

- Residents may need counselling to help them through emotional and relationship difficulties. Some problems may relate to past experience, others to present: either may be resolved through help which is focused on the individual or on her interactions with others.
- Remember always that residents need to feel a sense of control of what is happening to them. Staff should do all they can to enhance the reality and feeling of resident control.

WHERE TO LEARN MORE

A collection of nine booklets produced by the Centre for Policy on Ageing gives a very practical introduction to many of the issues in this chapter, and provides more detailed discussion of care tasks and skills:

Hodgkinson, J. (1988) *Home Work: Meeting the Needs of Elderly People in Residential Homes*, London: Centre for Policy on Ageing.

See also:

Worsley, J. (1989) *Taking Good Care: A Handbook for Care Assistants*, London: Age Concern England.

Two books written, respectively, by a physiotherapist and an occupational therapist offer practical detail on care tasks:

Hawker, M. (1985) *The Older Patient and the Role of the Physiotherapist*, London: Faber & Faber.
Hooker, S. (1981) *Caring for Elderly People: Understanding and Practical Help*, London: Routledge & Kegan Paul.

On counselling:

Scrutton, S. (1989) *Counselling Older People: A Creative Response to Ageing*, London: Edward Arnold.

Chapter Seven

LIVING TOGETHER: HELPING PEOPLE IN GROUPS

This chapter is concerned with things that happen when a number of individuals come together in a residential Home: it is about groups. The previous chapter emphasized ways of helping individuals, but the needs of individuals in a group situation cannot be neatly distinguished from the needs of groups as a whole. There are, therefore, many interrelationships between the concerns of the two chapters.

LIVING IN THE BUILDING

The physical characteristics of the building in which the Home exists will have strong influences on how people live and on the kinds of groups that are formed. There has been some discussion of basic aspects of this in Chapter 4. A small number of particularly significant research reports will be used here, briefly to summarize the most important issues.

Work in Local Authority Homes in Wales in the early 1970s (Slater and Lipman 1976) concluded that the then standard design of Home was deficient in a number of ways. These included:

- so-called bedsitting-rooms that were not large enough to be used as sitting-rooms and which did not permit flexible arrangements of furniture;
- toilets and bathrooms arranged in centralized blocks which minimized residents' opportunities to use them independently and in private;
- centralized communal dining areas and food preparation

areas to which residents did not usually have access;
- lengthy internal corridors that inhibited mobility and may well have contributed to spatial disorientation;
- unscreened personal accommodation, with doors opening directly into bedrooms.

Lipman and Slater proposed that designs should be based on an 'operational philosophy'. This centred on a belief that the physical settings in which people live should provide opportunities to be and remain independent, to maintain social contacts and to find privacy. This led them to proposals which they argued should

> enable residents (a) to exercise 'choice' *vis-à-vis* the use of their personal rooms as sitting rooms; (b) to maintain dignity *vis-à-vis* bathing and toileting; (c) to exercise 'independence' and 'self-care' by preparing at least some of their meals; (d) to retard 'deterioration' by minimizing the occurrence of spatial disorientation; and (e) to preserve 'privacy' by screening personal accommodation.
>
> (Lipman and Slater 1976: 13)

These themes were developed further by a study of 100 Homes in England (Willcocks *et al.* 1982). The researchers made a distinction between *public space,* such as lounges and dining rooms, and *private space,* such as bedrooms. They attempted a classification of Homes by physical type. At one extreme they described some as 'very integrated' where bedrooms, bathrooms and toilets were sited close to lounges and dining areas: typically, these tended to be larger, more recently built Homes. At the other extreme were Homes where clusters of lounges adjacent to dining-rooms were some distance from the bedrooms and bathrooms: these tended to be in smaller buildings and longer-established Homes.

The authors of this report argued that key elements in understanding the impact of internal design on the lives of residents are the ratio of private space to public space as well as the degree of integration or segregation of public and private areas. The study included interviews with residents and staff and, in a further report (Peace *et al.* 1982), it was argued that 'residential life is currently constructed socially, on an assumption that residents will be prepared to live out their lives in a largely public setting'.

In this sense, the authors argued, residential life is an 'unbalanced life' (p. 48), and they proposed a shift in the focus away from public and communal life towards the private and personal. Their study found that although some residents liked the traditional communal residential Home or the group-living arrangements, the majority would prefer to lead more individual lives. Their proposed solution was residential flatlets.

Clearly, then, the design of the Home affects how people live. The concentration of most studies has been on larger Local Authority Homes in which key issues have been the tendency for group-living or 'public' areas to be centrally situated, away from bedrooms, and the generally small bedroom areas which do not provide enough space or flexibility for people to live private lives in them for much of the day. In the search for practical solutions to the day-to-day difficulties which design failures in large Homes have caused, there has been a variety of developments in which smaller groups have been established within the larger Home. Generally, these have become known as group-living arrangements.

Actual practice and philosophy of such arrangements vary and there is considerable confusion about what group living is and why it is desirable. This is further complicated in the group Homes or family-group Homes which have developed, particularly in those where three or four people with mental handicaps live together in an 'ordinary house in an ordinary street'. The basic principle of small-group living in residential Homes for elderly people is that large Homes are divided into smaller areas in which groups of around eight to ten residents lead most of their daily life together. All the necessary facilities of bathroom, toilet, lounge, dining room and often a kitchen are within a small area close to bedrooms. The assumption is that a small group of eight or so people provides either a closer approximation to privacy or a more domestic, family-like environment, or both.

The approach puts emphasis on each resident being able to make a contribution to the daily needs of the group. Breakfast, for instance, is often prepared by residents, and facilities for making drinks and snacks are available. Often main meals are brought by heated trolley from a central kitchen and may be served by residents. In practice, this leads to problems and complications. Sometimes a small number of more able residents do (or feel that they do) most of the work each day. Staff may be assigned to each group in a Home: this may result in staff being thinly spread, may require higher staffing levels, and can cause difficulties if two staff are needed to lift a resident and one group may be left without help whilst assistance is given. During the busy times at the beginning of the mornings staff may be assisting residents to dress, changing soiled beds and trying to help with preparing food. There arise difficulties of trying to be in several places at once and, not least, of hygiene.

More fundamentally, studies of group-living arrangements have reported problems of personality clashes and arguments between residents. In the smaller group proximity to both those you like and those you dislike is increased: there is less chance to escape from difficult relationships and fewer people to choose from to make friends. In theory, there should be scope for people to visit other groups as they wish, but there is limited evidence that in practice residents living in small groups do move around: everything they need for survival tends to be provided in their own unit, which may nevertheless fail to offer all that they need for satisfaction.

There has been little substantial research into group living. What evidence there is suggests that such Homes may be a little better than traditionally organized Homes at preventing deterioration, may offer more intellectual stimulation and be more successful in supporting independent residents. On the other hand, they are less likely to improve residents functioning and are less successful in meeting the needs of moderately independent residents (Booth and Phillips 1987).

One other research report helps to put all these findings into context. Norman (1984) studied a number of Local Authority Homes, some based on a more traditional hotel-type model and others on the group-living model. At its best, the hotel model offers people the opportunity to live a private life in a comfortable bedsitting-room and to choose to mix with a variety of people in different lounge areas and to eat in a discrete and comfortable dining-room, with people they wish to be with. Yet it may also mean isolation and loneliness. At its best, the group living model offers more informal relationships with staff, greater opportunity to do daily living tasks and mix with a small group of friendly people.

Norman suggests that either type of Home can be run well to

provide the most important things – a wide degree of choice for residents about where they eat and sit, with whom they do these things and how much they do for themselves.

Some people have clearly found group-living arrangements a useful way of creating a resident-centred environment which provides, in large and often unsuitable buildings, a greater degree of choice, opportunity and personal control. There is also evidence that in some cases it has proved unsatisfactory for staff and residents. The important thing is that each group of staff and residents should have a chance themselves to think about and discuss how to make best use of the living space to provide what is best for them. In order to do so, a good understanding of group processes is essential for the residential worker to balance the wide range of competing and often conflicting needs to be found in the resident and staff groups.

UNDERSTANDING GROUPS

The last forty years or so have seen the development of a very considerable body of social work literature about how groups work and can be used to help people. Surprisingly, little of it has focused on elderly people. One reason for this is no doubt the general lack of interest in work with this group. More practically it may be related to the difficulties of getting older people together because of mobility problems and communication difficulties. There are, of course, many different approaches to group-work. These cannot be explored in detail here. Some general principles of group functioning can be set out, however.

How are groups made up?

It is quite common to talk about 'the residential group' as if it were a single, fixed entity. Life in Homes is, of course, much more complicated. Within a Home, there are many different groups which may shift and change frequently and which interlock and interrelate with each other and with groups outside. The staff group is itself made up of several groups, both formal (officers or management, care staff, domestic staff, etc.) and informal. These groups will have many links with similar groups in other Homes, community and family links and often connection with friends and relatives of the residents in the community. Similarly, residents form and re-form various groups in the lounges, at the dining tables, on outings, during organized activities, etc., as well as having their own outside links and membership of family and friendship groups in the community. The first thing to remember, then, is the complexity of the group interactions: residential workers do not work in a single group but in many groups.

The way in which any one group is made up or structured is influenced by several basic factors.

Membership

The membership of the group is its basic resource. A group of elderly people has a wealth of life experience and skills to draw from but each member also has a lifetime of habits, inhibitions and prejudices to contribute to the patterns of behaviour.

Roles

The roles played by people within the group give security and help to form the structure of behaviour. There are formal roles: care assistant, grandmother, cook, table-setter, officer-in-charge, etc. There are also informal roles such as conversation-starter, standard-setter, enabler, joker, etc.

Status

Groups will usually establish a 'pecking-order' in which its various members are seen to have status in particular situations. People do not necessarily hold the same status in different groups. A resident with good recall and local knowledge may take a leading role in a reminiscence discussion but may take a back seat for much of the rest of the time. The entry of a member of staff into a resident group discussion can strongly influence patterns of behaviour and relative status, and staff must be aware of how they can positively and negatively influence status and roles in groups of residents. Roles and status are of course, closely related and are usually also related to relative power (although not always so).

Communication

The communication patterns of groups tend to follow similar forms and are important indicators of status and role. Communication is largely verbal but also involves a wide range of actions which themselves indicate meanings. The way people sit, facial expression, gesture, or absence from the group convey messages.

Leadership

Each of the above contributes to the way leadership works in the group. Groups may have an acknowledged leader but often it is more appropriate to think in terms of actions which are designed to influence the behaviour of the whole group and which require the support of most of the group to have an effect. These leadership actions may be initiated by different people for different purposes or by a leading group within the larger group. In order to influence staff or resident behaviour, an understanding of how leadership actions influence decisions is essential. Change may only be possible with the tacit or explicit permission of the leader or leading group.

How do groups behave?

Once again, there are some complicated relationships between the ways in which groups behave and the ways individuals behave in groups. When people come together they influence each other to behave and reach decisions in ways they might not behave or decide individually. Some of the more important aspects of behaviour for the present purposes are as follows.

Territorial space

Groups often establish territorial space (as do most individuals). It is common in Homes for small groups to regard a particular area of the Home as their own and to resent intrusion. In practice this can cause problems for newcomers, although some groups are on the look-out for new members whom they see as 'their sort', and will welcome, for instance, someone from a familiar locality or of intellectual ability. Groups with an established space are often particularly resentful of elderly people who wander in a confused way and intrude on their territory. Staff should be aware of their right to choose their companions and special place but also of the rights of other people in the Home to enjoy its facilities. Sometimes a great deal of tact and skill is needed to enable newcomers to find their way into an established, territorial group or to encourage a more welcoming attitude to others.

Elites

In a similar way small groups of residents sometimes feel like and expect to be treated as elites: as special. Usually this tends to be based on intellectual ability: it may be those residents who are not suffering from dementia who tend to congregate together and expect to be treated differently. If this results in them providing mutual support and conversation, staying up late at night together, making tea for each other, etc., the results are likely to be positive. Staff should guard against rejection of less able, or less acceptable residents if that leads to a demand for unequal amounts of staff time and also resources.

Attraction and identification

The reasons why some people are attracted to each other and begin to identify with particular groups are many and varied. Not all people want to be actively involved in close-knit small groups. Some people tend to be withdrawn or separate from group activity: this may be from choice, either because they feel that they do not need the group or because they fear its influence or effect on them. An important task for the residential worker is to be aware of how groups within the Home are working to the benefit or detriment of individuals and to find ways of intervening to improve or offset those effects. It will be important, for instance, to assess whether a resident is apart from others because she wishes to take an 'audience' role or because she has been rejected, or because of depression or apathy. If the processes are understood, then a decision can be made about whether to intervene – but, above all, taking care not to usurp the personal authority and right to self-determination of each resident.

Scapegoating

Sometimes resident groups treat one member as a scapegoat. This is in some ways a method of achieving a greater degree of group cohesion and solidarity. If the group can come together in opposition to a common 'enemy', then this is likely to give members a feeling of strength as a group. Although this may have some positive value for those within the group, it often causes intolerable problems for the person who is scapegoated.

Sometimes this is a new member who may be seen as a threat to the existing situation and rejected in a closing of ranks. One answer to this will be to introduce a more positive view of the possibilities for new involvement. If the resident group is encouraged to rearrange into a wider range of different groupings then each resident will have the chance to choose amongst several groups in which to form different relationships. If residents are less heavily invested in a single group, they will be less likely to view other residents as a threat. It is especially important that staff do not become drawn into the pattern of scapegoating behaviour: it is often very tempting to join in what seems like mild mockery of slightly confused behaviour or eccentric characteristics, but it is unacceptable for staff to behave in this way.

Conflict

Groups can offer safety to their members but it is inevitable that conflicts will arise between people in the Home – not only amongst residents but also between staff and residents. The residential worker has available several methods of dealing with these situations. Some conflicts may even be stimulated – about practical improvements or decorations in the Home, for example. This may produce positive change: conflict may have a creative function. In more bitter, destructive situations the worker can be involved in clarifying what is really being said and making sure that both parties to an argument have understood what it is about. The worker can let each party to the conflict know that she can understand their points of view without being seen to take sides, and she can help to present each to the other in a more favourable light. Every opportunity should be taken to reduce ill feeling in a sensitive way that does not push the participants towards more entrenched positions.

Decision-making

Groups make decisions. These may not be the decisions that individuals would have made independently: together they are influenced by various factors such as leadership, group expectations as each member understands them, and predominant values in the group. Decision-making by resident groups, will be considered further in later discussion of participation and resident committees. Probably more important is the decision making of staff groups which is considered in the next chapter.

Apathy

A theme which runs throughout discussions of groups in residential Homes is that of apathy: perhaps more so in the care of elderly people. Apathy may be a response to group pressures: a way of reflecting how an individual feels within the group. It may also be a reflection of clinical depression or a realistic response to being in a powerless position. If people feel that whatever they do will have no effect on the world about them, they inevitably take no action and become apathetic: this has been called 'learned helplessness' (Seligman and Maier 1967). Once again, the worker has a responsibility to understand why a person appears to behave apathetically and to help if necessary.

Using groups

This very brief commentary on an enormously complicated subject gives some basic indication of common issues. For the residential worker there will be broadly two sorts of groups to consider: those which come together in the normal course of daily living and those which are created for a specific purpose, such as craftwork, entertainment, therapeutic discussion or activity.

Groups in daily living

This chapter has so far established that the physical environment strongly influences the groups that form in a Home and that a complex interrelationship of groups forms within the Home and with the outside world. One of the first principles is that residents should be able to choose who they sit with and relate to. If there are only two large lounges in a Home, or if there is a small group-living unit lounge for eight residents, each will place restrictions on choice and the nature of involvement with others. It is difficult to form a close, confiding friendship in a lounge with twenty other people listening. The more sitting spaces there are, the more people will be able to choose for themselves whom to talk to; staff may need to encourage residents to move around by offering different activities in different places. Often, residents feel they are expected to stay in one place and may need 'permission' to move around. This can be given explicitly or by example, encouragement and creating opportunities to do different things in different places.

A group can best grow from its point of mutual contact or common ground. Elderly people in Homes usually have local community contacts in common, and the worker should identify these and build on them. Simple 'talking points' from local newspapers or scrapbooks are easy to find. A good deal of work has been done recently on the use of reminiscence as a way of helping to orientate people and to provide discussion points; many aids to reminiscence now exist. If such approaches are used there are some common-sense rules to bear in mind: do not, for instance, offer pictures of the First World War to people whose most important life experiences were in the 1930s and 1940s: think about what will be meaningful to them. Remember also that not everyone enjoys looking back: the past can evoke sad memories as well as happy ones, so think about who will benefit and discuss it with them individually beforehand (and be prepared to talk to them afterwards if they are upset or distressed).

It is essential to pay attention to the outside links and groups with which residents are involved. In the resident group as a whole, the outside world can take on an appearance of unreality. If residents are very cut off from the outside there may be a tendency to cope with the pains of isolation by pretending that nothing outside the Home exists. This may account for exaggerated reactions to letters from outside, or excessive anxiety about visitors and obsessive reactions to lateness of arrival, etc. A link with the outside world may be a painful reminder of all that the residents are missing. The way to avoid this is to encourage much more active family and community links.

The local community can be brought in on many formal occasions – coffee mornings, fund-raising, concerts, etc. – which may lead to more informal contacts. If neighbours and other local residents feel free to call in at any time this will offer a wider range of relationships and choice to residents. The reverse is also true: residents should be able to get out to the local shops, church and clubs. Some will be able to go alone, others may need to be organized into group outings, but all should be encouraged to remain in touch with the reality of the outside world. Relatives should also be encouraged to take an active part in caring for their elderly parents. Sometimes relatives feel guilty about being unable to care and may see a suggestion that they should come into the residential Home to help as an accusation. Occasionally they project their guilt and become very hostile towards residential workers. Nevertheless, if they can be involved they provide useful additional contacts and stimulation for residents.

Some boundaries must be set on groups: members need to be sure of how far they can go. Too much intimacy in the group can be as frightening as too little interaction, and residents will feel safer with clear boundaries and limitations. Any limits should not be imposed in an authoritarian way. Being too dominating is likely to force the residents into child-like roles, with all the implications that has for dependent behaviour.

In being part of groups in the Home the residential worker should take part and assist individuals to develop relationships – if necessary, giving personal support to those who need encouragement to come further into the group. She should offer a flexible acceptance of the needs of both individuals and the group as a whole but should be able to remain sufficiently apart and separate from the group to preserve her own identity (that is, not get 'too involved'). She should also be able to set limits to protect individuals from too much group pressure or demands.

In their involvement in groups care workers may need assistance themselves in coping with the demands and dependence of residents. These can lead to often rewarding but sometimes stressful demands as people become close to each other. Groups of staff can support each other in dealing positively with the feelings that arise.

Groups with a Purpose

Three broad approaches to group-work with elderly people can be distinguished: those concerned with groups which are for leisure, education and activity; those concerned with self-help or participation in decision-making; and those which concentrate on individual growth, change or treatment in the group.

Leisure One valuable area for growth and stimulation at any age is in play. For the child, play fulfils certain psychological needs: exploration, movement and activity encourage learning and growth. Through play and imitation the child can explore and experiment with social roles and learn how it feels for others to be who they are. Play also has an important role in make-believe or fantasy. In playing alternative roles the child or adult can find new satisfactions and alternative compensations. Play, or perhaps quite simply *fun*, can fulfil similar functions for the elderly person. The use of music and movement sessions, whilst not acceptable to all residents, does provide some physical exercise, and singing stimulates memories as well as providing the actual satisfactions of the music itself and of the shared group activity. Other kinds of leisure activity – gardening, hobbies, handicrafts – should all be possible for those who want them. The growth of the University of the Third Age, providing educational opportunities, also offers a way of contributing to the lives of residents, both inside and away from the Home. Physical activity can often be best maintained through play and leisure pursuits, which have the added benefit of emotional satisfaction (they are fun to do) and intellectual stimulation (they keep the mind active).

Self-help and participation In the last fifteen years or so there has been considerable development in what might be called the self-help movement amongst elderly people. This ranges from those groups which have developed mainly to enable elderly people to share their skills and knowledge with each other or to join in leisure and educational groups, to those whose main purpose is overtly political. Task Force, a voluntary group working mainly in London, did a lot of work on developing community groups for elderly people. In a review of some of the projects in which Task Force had been involved, some of the aims of work with pensioners were described as giving them:

1. greater control
    (a) over the groups or clubs to which they belong;
    (b) over areas outside their groups which affect them e.g. access to local resources such as social services, welfare benefits;
    (c) over decisions which affect their lives
2. greater opportunity to develop their own creativity
3. greater opportunity to be and to feel useful
4. greater opportunity to get to know other people
5. greater opportunity to combat ageism.

(Buckingham *et al.* 1979)

These objectives should apply equally to elderly people in Homes. Elderly people should have the opportunity, together in groups, to influence decisions made about them and their daily lives and, through doing so, to feel useful and in control. Residential workers have tried various ways to encourage and enable this. Residents' committees have been established, flourished and faded as residents have come and gone. To maintain the impetus of resident participation in decision-making requires a high degree of commitment from staff as well as resident motivation. All this needs working at constantly: the rewards are worth the effort. Residents have a right and responsibility to be involved.

Growth, change and development Homes are not usually places in which intensive therapeutic groups are run. Often, staff do not have the time to contemplate such work and many staff have not had the training to be able to provide group-work of a kind to offer a therapeutic approach to individual growth and development. There is, however, potential for such work, properly planned and with appropriately limited goals.

'Reality orientation' has become a commonly used expression in Homes but is not always adequately understood or used. It describes a way of stimulating and responding to residents which can assist them to recover skills, help them keep in touch with the world and reduce confused behaviour. There are two types of reality orientation:

- In twenty-four-hour reality orientation, staff respond consistently to residents by giving them information which helps to orientate them. They use the resident's names frequently, refer to the place, time, day, weather, etc., whenever possible. Labels and notices may be used to remind them where to go, what is for lunch, or what day it is: there is a consistent approach to reinforcing practical realities.
- In classroom reality orientation, small groups of residents meet for a more systematic teaching-style session, perhaps naming objects, matching pictures to words and repeating key information.

There is mixed research evidence about the effectiveness of reality orientation. Certainly, it seems clear that where staff are consistent and reinforce current information about the environment this does help to reduce disorientation and offset the effects of memory loss. The use of notices and labels is of more debatable value: they may contribute to making the Home look institutional and they *must* be kept up to date. A clear sign that it is Tuesday 5th on Wednesday 6th can only be confusing!

One general issue confirmed in several research studies of group-work is the need to involve all staff in planning because of the possibility, otherwise, of conflict and confusion. It may be that change in a Home is as likely to come about from staff training and changes in staff attitudes as from the group-work itself.

One useful, small-scale study attempted to distinguish the main themes and models of group-work with elderly people. The first was called the 'Here and Now' model, based on the approach of the learning theorists which suggests that focusing on the past or the future encourages people to avoid dealing with the present. The second – the 'There and Then' model – emphasizes the past and the importance of using the life-review approach. Comparing two groups, each using one of these models, the authors concluded that each can be useful for some people (Ingersoll and Silverman 1978). Considerable skill and experience is needed, however, to determine which resident is most likely to benefit from a particular group.

This brief introduction to some issues in working with groups of elderly people should confirm the need for residential workers to be skilled in helping groups to function effectively in a range of areas:

- using the physical space creatively to provide people with a choice of groups with whom to mix;
- helping day-to-day groups of residents that form naturally in the Home to work to everyone's advantage;
- ensuring that residents can take part in a range of leisure, activity and education groups if they want to;
- using groups to enable residents to take part in decision-making about the life of the Home;
- providing therapeutic, group counselling or reality orientation groups where necessary and appropriate.

MENTAL DISORDER IN THE RESIDENTIAL GROUP

One of the most difficult aspects of working with elderly people in the enclosed setting of the Home is coping with the behaviour of people with a mental disorder. Unusual, wandering, demanding, challenging or aggressive behaviour will be difficult for both staff and residents to cope with. Such behavioural difficulties can arise for many reasons.

The most common disorders in Homes are depression and forms of dementia. Probably between a third and two-thirds of residents in many Homes suffer from some form of mental disorder. The worker will need to be alert to the signs of change in behaviour. The first step, when behaviour does change or when unexplained physical changes occur, should be to seek skilled assessment and treatment for the resident.

Depression is a term which is often used loosely. It can mean unhappiness or generally feeling sad or out of sorts. It may refer to a reaction to an important loss: bereavement and grief. It may also be used to describe profound mood changes which occur unexpectedly and for no immediately obvious reason: this is known as endogenous depression. A resident suffering from endogenous depression may lose weight and appetite and may be restless, often during the night. Activity usually slows down, although some people do become agitated and over-active. It is quite common for the apathy and reduced activity to be accompanied by some disorientation and reduced awareness of reality. This can be mistaken for the signs of dementia with the risk that proper assessment and treatment will not be sought.

Some of the elements of dementia, or chronic brain failure, were discussed in Chapter 2. Psychiatric and psychological textbooks should be consulted for a full understanding. Gray and Isaacs (1979: 16) have written particularly helpfully and summarize the main manifestations of brain failure as:

(i)   a tendency to commit errors;
(ii) a failure to perceive errors;
(iii) a failure to comprehend the consequences of errors.

The consequence of this in Homes can be unpleasant. Often brain failure leads to lack of attention to clothing and personal hygiene, and to not going to the toilet or going in inappropriate places. It is associated, for some, with incessant wandering, searching behaviour which intrudes on others, often to the extent of going into private rooms, removing possessions or sleeping in beds. Occasionally, there may be violent or aggressive behaviour or other unacceptable behaviour as inhibitions are reduced. All these affect the lives of other residents and disrupt the patterns of group living.

There are, however, some ways in which the residential worker can organize and behave to reduce the difficulties.

The balance of the group

The debate about whether people with dementia should be integrated with intellectually able residents or segregated, either in separate Homes or into different groups within a Home, has gone on for a long time. It remains inconclusive. There are two broad aspects to the debate: whether it is desirable or not to separate out some people and whether it is practicable or not to do so. The first is a question of attitudes and values, the second one of skills and resources: but the two are hard to separate.

One of the most substantial research studies of the mixing of confused and lucid residents concluded that a policy of full integration of impaired and more able residents should be pursued. However, it suggested that, 'The need for a balance of confused and lucid residents should be recognized. No Home should be expected to care for more than 30% suffering moderate or severe confusion' (Evans *et al.* 1981). The research points to the importance of staffing resources, both numbers and skills, and to the need for a balance of physically able people in a Home. A later study (Norman 1987a) suggests that there is general agreement that some dementia sufferers are too disruptive, aggressive or uncooperative to be given adequate care in a residential setting. The author points out, however, that we do not really know what it is that hospital wards provide for such people that Homes cannot provide.

If people with and without dementia are to live together in Homes then decisions do need to be made about balances: of staff resources to resident needs; of confused to lucid residents; and of physically less able to more able residents. Some degree of difficult behaviour may be manageable without placing unfair stress on staff and other residents, but to do so takes up staff time which is therefore not available to do other things: resident support, promoting activities, etc. A careful balance can quickly be upset by the addition of one resident whose behaviour is difficult: it is prudent for a Home to retain some spare capacity for such times.

Of course, your attitude to integration or segregation of confused residents may be different if someone has just wandered into your room and removed half your clothing from the wardrobe or has lain in your bed and wet it. For residents, in other words, this is not an academic policy debate and many more able residents do find such behaviour disruptive and distressing. It is a very difficult balance to strike.

Talking and listening

Many of the problems that arise relate to difficulties of memory. Memory is actually a lot of different things: not, as is often thought, a single thing which, like a muscle, will get stronger if it is exercised. In order to remember, the brain needs the ability to *receive* information, to *retain* and store it and then to *recall* it when it is needed. Changes in the brain resulting from dementia, or perhaps a stroke, can affect one or more of these abilities.

The worker can help in various ways:

- Prompting can assist with recall: finding a variety of references to things associated with the subject may help the elderly person to retrieve the information from memory.
- If they have difficulty in retaining information a notepad or diary can sometimes help. More simply, staff need to have the patience and understanding to recognize that simple instructions or information may need to be repeated frequently to some people.
- The ability to actually receive information may be affected by many things: sensory changes as well as brain changes. It will not be enough to use words to tell people something: gestures, pictures or actually showing them may need to be added to the words.

Reference was made earlier to reality orientation as one way of helping residents to remain in contact with the world and current events. A consistent approach to using the resident's name and referring to events, circumstances and surroundings will help people to stay in touch with reality. Sometimes the use of recall and reminiscence can also help to remind people of who they are and assist in keeping them alert in the present. Remember, however, that most of us indulge in 'careful forgetting': we choose not to remember some uncomfortable things. The capacity of the memory to select things out can be necessary to people, so be alert for uncomfortable memories.

Talking and listening to residents who appear confused is essential: many apparently irrational behaviours are for a reason. Wandering, for example, may really be a searching for a former home, or be associated with times of day: giving people familiar tasks, such as peeling vegetables before lunch or washing up after a meal may distract and help to fix their location in their minds. Most people in any new situation 'wander' in the sense that they look around to get their bearings. New residents may have coped in their familiar home surroundings but may be disorientated and will need time and help (by, for instance, talking, accompanying them on walks around the Home and grounds, etc.) to adjust.

Distraction or confrontation

Some people with dementia are able to carry on an apparently normal conversation on a superficial, social level about familiar topics such as their family or the weather. They confabulate: fill in gaps in their memory with plausible stories. Pursuing the conversation will produce clues about the extent of the confusion ('I really must go now, I've left the baby on the draining-board').

Whatever the extent of confusion there will be occasions when workers will be faced with the need to respond to irrational conversation or behaviour: waiting for parents who died thirty years ago; setting off to find a home and children all long gone; a stubborn insistence that money handed to a daughter has been stolen by someone in the Home, etc. It is rarely helpful to confront the behaviour directly: to the resident, their perception of the situation is real. It is usually better to divert or distract. If someone is setting off to look for a former house it may be enough to point out that it is cold outside and propose having lunch first. If this does not work then actually going out for a walk with the resident can offer other distractions: a walk in the park, stopping off at the shops, etc., before returning to the Home.

Arguing with a confused resident about whether or not her husband is dead can only be distressing and lead to problems. Far better to change the subject, suggest going for breakfast, discuss the weather or talk about which clothes to put on. On the other hand, it may only add to the confusion if staff respond as if the resident's perception is correct. The important thing is to hear what people are saying: to look for any factual basis in what they are asking or seeking. It may arise from discomfort, from a misunderstood conversation or from unhappiness; the worker ought to be able to help with all of these.

The basic principles of practice with elderly people with mental disorder can be summarized:

1 Be alert for physical and intellectual changes and seek skilled assessment, advice and treatment from a psychiatrist and/or psychologist as appropriate.
2 Talk to people who appear confused and disorientated: listen to what they have to say and be alert for any meanings behind apparently odd behaviour.
3 Respond courteously and do not try to deal rationally with irrational behaviour: distraction is better than confrontation. But also try not to collude with irrationality.

Helping elderly residents, especially those with a degree of brain failure involves taking some risks. A more detailed discussion of risk is therefore essential, especially in relation to people with mental disorder.

RISK TAKING

Risk can be made into a complicated concept. Some people, especially in the fields of commercial insurance and of hazards in the workplace, have put a lot of time into doing so and some have made a successful living from it. Risk is a word we use casually in everyday conversation with several meanings and it will be helpful, without becoming too complex, to define it more clearly before proceeding to consider what risk-taking means.

There are two elements to risk. First, it is an expression of probability or likelihood. It is used to mean that there is a chance, probability or possibility that something will happen. Second, risk is usually used to mean that there is a chance of something unpleasant or harmful occurring. The two main elements, then, are *likelihood* and *loss*, damage or harm. This is an approach which stresses the variation that occurs in events (you cannot be sure what will happen)and their potential costs for people.

A slightly different way of thinking about it is to consider the relationship between situations or events and their outcomes. We can only begin to protect against risks if we have some idea of how likely something is to happen and relate that to the factors that may bring it about. It is useful, therefore, to distinguish between hazards and dangers. A hazard is anything – an action, event, lack or circumstance – which introduces or increases the probability that some harm will occur. A danger is the outcome that is feared. In this sense, a loose carpet or wet floor are hazards because they introduce the danger of slipping and falling.

To make sense of risk, then, it is necessary to be clear about what we fear may go wrong (the danger), what it is that makes that outcome a possibility (the hazard) and how probable the outcome is. If we can do this it becomes possible to think more clearly about whether the risk can be managed – by reducing or removing the hazards to lessen the likelihood of something going wrong or reducing the extent of actual damage if it does go wrong.

Safe or safe enough?

The other side of the risk coin is safety. A precise definition of safety would relate it to a situation in which there was no chance of harm: no risk. But in the real world there is no totally risk-free situation. In practice, safety is usually used to mean that the risks are judged to be negligible or acceptable (they are not great enough to worry about). Safe therefore commonly means 'safe enough'. Deciding whether something is safe or that the known risks are acceptable depends on being able to do two things:

1 Estimate the risks: how likely is it that harm will occur?
2 Evaluate the risks: how serious will the consequences be?

When this has been done two further decisions become possible:

3 Can the likelihood be changed/reduced: what can be done about the hazards?
4 Is the balance between likelihood and the severity of the consequences acceptable?

169

This seems fairly straightforward but, unfortunately, most human situations are difficult to predict and there is plenty of evidence that people are poor estimators of risk. Subjective estimates of risk are influenced by many things: the type of risk, the extent to which it is seen to be controllable, and whether or not people can imagine the effect of the outcomes. Such factors will all affect attitudes to risk. Some dangers, for example, are so unpleasant to contemplate that people may behave as if they do not exist. Fire in Homes is one example of this: there is a danger that staff and residents will resist precautions because the consequences are too horrific to think about. Attitudes to risk are also affected by the general view of the world that people hold: some take a pessimistic view and are reluctant to take risks; others enjoy risk-taking and consciously gamble.

Attitudes to risk-taking are, therefore, strongly influenced by personal belief and social context. Risk-taking has commonly been advocated as a desirable part of residential life for elderly people. In reality this does not seem to mean that residents should be exposed to hazards and danger: there is nothing desirable about living life 'in danger'. It does seem to mean that residents should be able to make choices about their own lives, even if that exposes them to hazards and dangers. The right of the individual should take precedence.

In residential Homes it is rarely quite so simple. The right of one elderly person to put herself at risk often exposes others to risk. Staff will feel responsible and may be held responsible by others for the safety of residents. This is complicated: they will be expected to behave responsibly towards residents and to do what is reasonable to protect the rights of all involved. The residential worker should be concerned with five key factors in enabling residents to make choices and decide about risks:

1 Creating a range of choices: if there are more choices available, then the elderly person may be attracted to a less dangerous option.
2 Extending the knowledge of residents about the choices open to them: people cannot choose if they do not know what is available.
3 Contributing to the resident's ability – emotional or intellectual – to decide, by discussion and clarification.

170

4 Helping people to live with the consequences of decisions: if something does go wrong the worker can help to reduce or repair the damage.

5 Dealing with the impact of the decision on other people.

It is the last of these that tends to loom the largest in communal living. If one resident chooses to smoke in the bedroom, that puts everyone else at risk. If she decides to go out and is involved in an accident, staff may be blamed and, at the very least, will feel guilty. If she wanders on the road and causes an accident, others may be hurt or damaged.

Risk-taking is related to the balancing of freedom and safety of individuals and of the whole group. It is this balance which is at the heart of the residential work task with elderly people. A degree of risk – of exposure to hazard and uncertainty – is an inevitable part of life. It is important for workers and residents to discuss and agree on acceptable levels of risk: on what is safe enough for them. That should be discussed and agreed by senior managers to ensure support for the practical decisions that have to be made.

For the residential worker, the best protection lies in a clear agreement about good practice, recorded in writing and agreed with those in authority. This agreement should be based on an objective assessment of the risks and of whether they can reasonably be reduced by removing or reducing hazards.

There has to be an acceptance that life cannot be *completely safe*, but each resident has a right to assume the environment has been made *reasonably safe*.

STRANGERS IN THE HOME

Another important impact on the residential group is that of those who come into the Home on a temporary basis, either for daily care and support, returning home in the evening, or for short periods of perhaps one or two weeks. Such temporary visitors can be intrusive into the lives of permanent residents, can make unpredicted demands on staff time and often have a major effect on how groups behave in the Home.

Research studies of short-term care in Homes have suggested that there are problems for both residents and Homes which may far outweigh the benefits (Allen 1983). The needs of short-stay elderly residents tend to be very different from those of long-stay residents and may not be satisfactorily met in a Home where most people are living on a permanent basis. Research suggests that short-stay care may be most successful in a Home which specializes in providing for short-stay residents only or where one wing or unit of a larger Home is turned over to that form of care.

There are specific difficulties. Short stays, especially when they are on a rotating or phased basis, may cause or exacerbate confusion. It was earlier shown that admission to a Home can be damaging, especially to the most frail elderly people, and may even lead to death for some. A series of admissions is potentially even more dangerous. The main beneficiaries of short-term care tend to be the carers of elderly people in the community: short stays provide, in other words, respite rather than rehabilitation.

Elderly people seek short-term care for three broad groups of reasons.

The first category is when the main purpose is to provide respite or relief for the people who provide care in the community. Often, this is to enable family or friends to take an annual holiday or attend to family matters, but increasingly it is being used to give carers a routine break to give them a rest. Usually, it is assumed that both the elderly person and the carers will benefit from a break from routine and each other. There is, however, the potentially confusing effect for the elderly person simply of change or of going for a 'holiday' in a Home which will have little in common with what most people usually regard as a holiday break.

Second, some short stays provide assessment and rehabilitation. In practice, this tends to be a minor element of most stays. Few Homes have the staff resources or other professional capacity to carry out full assessment, let alone to offer assistance in the relearning or development of skills which will enable an elderly person to return to live more successfully in the community. But it can be done: there is great potential if a scheme is properly resourced and organized.

Third, short stays are often the result of emergency admissions. Different agencies mean different things by 'emergency' but there is evidence that a high proportion of admissions do occur in emergency. It does not seem to be common practice to review circumstances immediately on admission. There is a strange gap in social work thinking; no social worker should admit a child to care without holding an immediate case conference, yet often elderly people are admitted with relatively little forward planning. There should always be immediate attention to the future: the space in the community can rapidly close up behind an elderly person if steps are not taken at once to preserve the position.

The actual time spent in short-term stays and the patterns of provision vary widely. Stays range from occasional or one-off placements arranged well in advance, through frequent but irregular placements, to planned periods of care arranged on a regularly repeated basis. These last are known as rotating or phased care arrangements and have been becoming increasingly common.

Short stays have great potential to offer a variety of rewards to the different people involved. If the stays are to be used effectively, some basic issues need attention:

1 They may be best provided in specialist Homes or units of established Homes. This is less intrusive on permanent residents and enables the regime to be geared to the special needs of short-stay residents. It has sometimes been argued that day-care or short-stay residents bring in news of the 'outside world' and provide interest and stimulation. This may sometimes be so, but if permanent residents need such news and stimulation there are many other creative ways of arranging community involvement.

2 They should be planned and purposeful. If the purpose is respite, that should be clear: but the potential for rehabilitation should be explored and opportunities to develop skills be taken wherever possible. This implies appropriate training and skills for staff and the involvement of a variety of professionals: physiotherapists, occupational therapists, etc. The longer-term plan for the elderly resident should be considered. Rotating care may be offered because the family wish to continue providing a home until death, but it may also be a phased admission – a way of providing relief until a permanent place can be found. It should be clear which is the case: the latter may be more appropriately provided in a long-stay Home, the former in a specialist, short-stay Home.

3 There should be help for the elderly person to cope with the changes of environment and to reduce the stress of moving. Continuity can be maintained by invitations to events or just

to tea in between stays in the Home. Keeping in touch by letter and cards on birthdays and Christmas can also keep up a useful link.

4 Finally, short stays should be approached with caution: they can be disturbing and confusing for the elderly person and intrusive on permanent residents. If planned, well organized and in the right place for the right people, they can be a useful contribution to clear, longer-term planning for the individual.

THE NEEDS OF BLACK AND ETHNIC MINORITY ELDERLY PEOPLE

Reference has been made throughout the book to the importance of taking account of cultural and ethnic differences. Stress has, in any case, been placed on allowing for differences between people. The issue of race, cultural and ethnic difference, must take an important place in any consideration of how to run residential Homes.

A report by the Standing Conference of Ethnic Minority Elderly Citizens (1988) stresses that ethnicity must be seen to be a source of cohesion, identity and strength which is as important for elderly people as it is for younger people. The report refers to the extent of physical and mental illness amongst elderly members of black and ethnic minority communities, often untreated because of poor communication with medical practitioners and other professionals. It points also to the fact that they are often worse off financially than indigenous elderly people for a variety of reasons. Ageing therefore involves, for these people, financial and emotional insecurity.

The report argues that, for many, the traditional approach to residential and other forms of care may be inappropriate and unacceptable. The idea of small Homes, within or close to the community is suggested as more appropriate. The report recommends that, in the short term, space and accommodation should be made available for group arrangements in a Home where properly trained staff of the same cultural and linguistic background as the elderly person should be attached or appointed. In the longer term, it proposes that thought should be given to the financing of voluntary initiatives by the communities themselves;

174

to the allocation of space in Local Authority Homes with appropriate staff for the different community groups; and to ensuring that all Homes have staffing to reflect the cultural diversity of the community.

This particular piece of work was focused on London. There are many parts of Britain where ethnic minorities form a very small proportion of the community, but all Homes should give time and thought – as part of their staff recruitment and training in particular – to meeting the special needs of minority groups.

HELPING PEOPLE IN GROUPS: KEY ISSUES

This chapter has considered issues surrounding the provision of help to groups of elderly people. In particular, it has stressed:

- The need to be aware of the influence of the design and physical features of the Home on the ways groups come together and behave.
- The complexity and variety of group relationships: there is not one residential group but interrelated and interlocking staff and resident groups which connect in many ways with the outside world.
- Workers can help residents to live more satisfyingly by assisting with relationships in groups during the process of day-to-day life, but also by establishing groups for special or specific purposes (education, leisure, personal development and counselling, etc.).
- A major feature in many Homes is the extent of mental disorder which pervades the group experience: staff can help by ensuring that proper assessment is carried out and by seeking to hear and respond to the needs and wishes of all residents.
- Encouraging and enabling people to choose their own lifestyle involves taking risks. Attitudes to risk are influenced by many subjective factors. Workers should take every reasonable step to ensure that residents live in a safe environment but enable them to exercise choice in a responsible manner, even if that involves taking risks. The balance between freedom and safety involves complex decisions about the needs, rights and responsibilities of groups and of the individuals within them.

- Group living can be significantly affected by short-term and day care. The intrusion of 'strangers' into the daily lives of permanent residents can be disturbing and unsatisfactory for everyone concerned. Care should be taken to plan for the most effective use of resources: the right people should be in the right place. This may mean specialist facilities, staffed appropriately to meet the different needs of short- and long-term residents and people who need day-care help.
- The needs of black and other ethnic minority elderly people should be centrally considered and appropriate provision made. This may need to include special accommodation for people from similar cultural backgrounds and should certainly include staff to reflect local cultural and ethnic diversity.

WHERE TO LEARN MORE

On the subject of design and physical structure Peace *et al.* (1982) and Norman (1984), referred to in the text, provide a good range of debate.

On group living:

Douglas, T. (1986) *Group Living: The Application of Group Dynamics in Residential Settings*, London: Tavistock Publications.

On mental disorder, Gray and Isaacs (1979) and Norman (1987a), referred to in the text, are useful. An excellent collection of short papers gives wide-ranging background:

Gearing, B., Johnson, M. and Heller, T. (eds) (1988) *Mental Health Problems in Old Age*, New York: John Wiley & Sons.

On risk:

Brearley, P. *et al.* (1982) *Risk and Ageing*, London: Routledge & Kegan Paul.

On short-term care:

Allen, I. (1983) *Short Stay Residential Care for the Elderly*, London: Policy Studies Institute.

On black and other ethnic minority groups, the Standing Conference of Ethnic Minority Citizens (1988) report is mentioned in the text. Also valuable is:

Bhalla, A. and Blakemore, K. (1981) *Elders of the Minority Ethnic Groups*, London: AFFOR.

Finally, a useful, short report on a project to improve quality of life which gives some interesting insights into staff-group reactions in particular is:

Potter, P. and Wiseman, V. (1989) *Improving Residential Practice: Promoting Choice in Homes for Elderly People*, London: National Institute for Social Work.

Chapter Eight

GOOD LIVES AND GOOD JOBS: BRINGING IT ALL TOGETHER

So far this book has been about the residential work task primarily from a resident-focused point of view: with creating an environment in which elderly people can be helped to lead a satisfying, enabling life. But those tasks can also be seen from the point of view of organization and management: in relation to how all the necessary work activities of staff can be brought together and managed. This chapter looks at issues mainly from the staff point of view.

It is at this point that some of the differences between public- and independent-sector Homes become most obvious. The basic principles of caring for people and creating a good home are the same whatever the ownership of the Home. But there are some significant organizational differences which have to be taken into account. For instance, for the manager of an individual Home there will be differences in day-to-day tasks (such as payment of wages, involvement in recruitment and selection of staff) as well as in accountability and responsibility (responsibility to a private proprietor rather than to an elected Council; accountability to a Local Authority inspector as well as proprietor, senior manager, etc.). The broad principles which are discussed here are generally applicable; as far as possible the clumsy repetition of the 'yes-but factor' (but in private Homes; but in the voluntary sector, etc.) will be avoided. Its relevance should, however, be borne in mind throughout.

The most significant resource for helping residents is the staff. It is essential that they work together as a team, with a clear idea of what they are seeking to achieve and why. The Head of Home is the key person who will influence the effectiveness of staff and who will need skills to organize, lead, motivate, plan, supervise, etc. These are some of the skills of management. Before discussing management skills in more detail, it will be helpful to recap on the actual tasks to be done.

THE TASKS TO BE DONE

There are a lot of ways of looking at this. The tasks for the Head of Home are different from those of care assistants, cooks and others. In a broad sense all of the tasks are concerned with three main areas of work: the building, the day-to-day business of running and making a home within it, and providing personal care and other help to the individuals who live there. The major groups of tasks will be related to:

- *The building*: ensuring that it exists in the first place, that its design is appropriate and that it is in the right place; subsequently maintaining it and adapting it as needs change. In Local Authority Homes much of this may be outside the control of the Head of Home. It will usually be dealt with by Maintenance, Capital Projects or Property Services Sections. In many private Homes much of this responsibility remains with the manager of the Home, offering greater control but additional demands on time which might otherwise be spent with residents. Whatever the arrangements, it should be possible for staff and residents to influence desirable changes to the building and to obtain an immediate response to the need for repairs.
- *Equipping, furnishing and decorating it*: at this point, two related factors emerge – the importance of residents having a say in the furniture and surroundings they want but also the need to balance the needs and wishes of staff and residents where these differ. One example is the provision of special baths. Some staff and residents insist on hoists and other adapted or special facilities. Others say they hate them and want ordinary baths. Personal preference is important but so is being clear about whose preferences take precedence. Residents have a right to choice of how they will bathe: staff have a right to avoid back strain!

- *Keeping it clean*: on the whole, domestic staff tend to be responsible for keeping the building clean; care staff tend to be responsible for helping residents to keep themselves and their clothing clean. Cooks have a vital responsibility for keeping kitchens clean. All have a shared responsibility for promoting hygiene and cleanliness.
- *Provisions and catering*: making sure that food, cleaning materials, soap and other personal toiletries are available.
- *Staffing*: the extent to which senior staff of the Home carry responsibility for recruitment, selection, training, paying wages, etc. varies widely, especially between public and private sectors. Responsibility for ensuring that the Home is staffed by the appropriate number of people, with the proper skills and at the right times, has to fall primarily on the Head of Home.
- *Personal care and Homemaking*: final responsibility for the tasks associated with looking after people falls to the Head of Home but many of the actual tasks fall to the care staff: assistance with washing, dressing, bathing, feeding, moving around, etc.
- *Administration and accounting*: all of these tasks require a system that administers the Home: that makes sure everything happens in the right place at the right time. They also require a system of financial accounting. It is part of the complexity of the role of a Head of Home that she is involved in managing as well as in residential social work, home-making and personal care. There are, however a variety of arrangements for managing these elements of the task. Homes may, for instance, employ an administrative head and a head of care, housekeeper, or some variant on these.
- *Living with the world outside*: informally, contact with the world outside happens in many ways. There is also a formal responsibility, carried by the Head of Home, for liaison with other agencies, contact with suppliers, links with churches and other community groups, dealing with inspectors, etc.

That, then, is the range of tasks: maintaining an appropriate building, running the business and helping people in a homely environment. The Head of Home, as the manager, must take the responsibility for keeping all of these together.

ON BEING A MANAGER

The Head of Home has to be many things, but especially a residential social worker, an administrator and a manager. To summarize briefly, as a residential social worker she is responsible for group and individual well-being and welfare; as an administrator, for the practical and clerical tasks of running the business; but as a manager, for the leadership and effectiveness of the Home as a whole organization. The manager has to plan services and make sure that they reach residents in the most suitable and effective way. The manager's main resources are the physical 'plant' (buildings and furnishings) and the staff.

Management is concerned with all the things that need to be done to make sure the purposes of the Home are achieved. There are some particularly important elements to the manager's role:

1 understanding and responding to the 'customer';
2 setting consistent, achievable goals derived from clear values;
3 taking action to achieve those goals;
4 making sure people have clear responsibilities for defined tasks;
5 training and motivating staff;
6 communicating and informing effectively;
7 monitoring what is (or is not) being achieved;
8 adapting quickly to change when necessary.

Particularly influential in social services agencies in recent years has been *In Search of Excellence* (Peters and Waterman 1982). This stresses, amongst other things, the importance of strong central direction and of the people within organizations listening to and responding to customers and encouraging maximum individual autonomy for staff. Particular stress is also put on organizations being responsive to change. Effective organizations are said to be ones which are flexible, have clear objectives based on explicit values and which value people.

Values and objectives

Values should be made explicit so that they can be discussed by staff. Only when they are spelled out clearly can their practical implications be debated and understood. The right to privacy, for example, may involve two elderly people choosing to sleep together; the right to choice may lead to a confused resident wandering away from the Home and being at risk of an accident or of getting lost. These, and similar issues, need to be thought about in relation to basic values: senior staff must take a lead in clarifying and discussing them.

When values are mutually understood and agreed they can be used as the basis for setting goals. These will include longer-term, overall objectives for the Home as a whole. They will also include shorter-term goals for the unit, or parts of it (e.g. to introduce a key-worker system; to devise a new system of recording; to replace uncomfortable beds; to make links with community groups, etc.). These may be set at a meeting of staff, or staff and residents and supporters of the Home at a periodic review meeting which can consider what has been achieved in the previous period and what to do next. All goals should be consistent with the agreed values and made known to all staff, who should have an opportunity to discuss and understand them.

Goals will also be set by and for residents. These should also be consistent with the agreed values and appropriate to the stated purpose and objectives of the Home.

Believing in excellence, believing in people

Traditionally, management literature has stressed the importance of leadership to effective working. The manager has been seen as being concerned with control and co-ordination. Various models of leadership have been described which place the manager in a central role of leading, motivating, controlling and co-ordinating their staff. Clearly, some control and co-ordination are essential to running an organization. There must be budgets, financial control systems, formal ways to reward and evaluate staff performance, arrangements for planning and goal-setting, and systems for monitoring whether tasks are being properly carried out.

However, if the Head of Home takes a very central, directive role, there is a likelihood that this will actually interfere with the development of a commitment amongst staff to the values and goals of the unit. These may tend to be seen as the property of the manager: the more so the more directive the role she takes. An effective system is likely to be one in which all members of staff have some autonomy themselves to take action to further the aims of the Home. The important principle is to establish a clear set of targets and ways of operating, based on an understanding of agreed values, and then to enable staff to develop their own patterns and relationships within their particular sphere of work.

To do this requires confidence on the part of the manager and a belief in the purposes and in the staff who work for her. This is not to suggest that people be left to their own devices: rather the opposite. They should be encouraged to use their initiative and skills within clear guidelines and guidance. But managers should believe in the approach. In a follow-on to *In Search of Excellence*, Peters, writing with Austin (1985: 101) comments, 'The heart of quality is not technique. It is a commitment by management to its people and products – stretching over a period of decades and lived with persistence and passion – that is unknown in most organizations today.'

Most management theory has developed in business organizations. A commitment to people is central to social work but is rather different in the context of social services management, although the idea of client or user as customer translates easily. One central issue in Homes is that the manager must value both staff and residents and must take account of the individual needs of each. On occasions, these will be in tension with each other. Staff, for instance, need a rest from often hard physical work. They appreciate a private staff rest-room away from residents: yet this is not something found in a domestic household.

An important role for the manager is therefore to balance these potentially conflicting groups of needs to ensure a happy staff group and satisfied residents. This is often challenging and demanding and the key, again, lies in agreed values which can help to explain and justify decisions to either or both groups.

Creating a culture

The most important thing about a Home is how it feels to be there, for visitors, staff or residents. It is the 'atmosphere' – the ambience, the culture. All of these words can be used to describe the way people behave and respond to the Home as a whole. Although there should be a shared responsibility, it will be the Head of Home who holds it all together.

Ideally, the staff of a Home should work together as a team, co-operating in achieving the agreed aims. An important way of achieving a feeling of working as a team is regular, purposeful meetings. There may be different groups of staff who need to work together as a team on any given task. Teams may come together for a very specific, short-term task (e.g. planning a fund-raising event or developing a new application form) or for permanent tasks (kitchen staff, care staff, senior officers, etc.). There will need to be different types of meetings of these various groups.

The senior managers group should meet weekly. It is easy to slip into the habit of communicating through message books and notes: this is not sufficient to maintain a consistent approach to running a Home. It is quite possible, for instance, for staff on one shift to work to a consistent approach to toileting for a group of residents but for another shift to work to another system. At this very basic level face-to-face meetings are essential. There should also be time for the different groups of staff – care, domestic, unit-living teams, etc. – to meet together routinely. This also requires some careful planning of rotas and a commitment to the importance of talking to each other.

Meetings should have a time and date, planned in advance and communicated to those who need to be there. They should have an agenda, and a note of decisions should be kept. Effective meetings have a clear purpose and keep to the point. They do not need to take a long time: just long enough to do the business in hand.

All the staff in the Home need to understand and agree with the basic aims and approaches. Some meetings of all staff will there-fore be necessary. The frequency of these will vary depending on the size of the Home. Sometimes, meetings will need to be held quite often, especially if there are major changes or developments or when the Home is first starting. Such meetings may have to focus on development and training as well as practical issues. In established Homes, they may be held less often and be more concerned with current business.

Most groups have potential for conflict. Some of the main causes of conflict are:

1 Where people have different or inadequate information and therefore understand things differently. This can be overcome by good communication, through notices, good written records, good hand-overs between shifts, and concise, to-the-point meetings.

2 Where people are trying to achieve different things. Sometimes this is because they have different basic values: some, for instance, feel that elderly people have worked hard all their lives and are entitled to have things done for them, others believe they are best helped to help themselves. If there is such a basic disagreement it will inevitably lead to dispute and radically differing practices. Often people have 'hidden agendas': their real wishes and objectives are different from the ones they say they have. This becomes obvious from the way they actually behave, and suspicion and disagreement result. The way to deal with this is through clarity of goals, discussion and training. Sometimes people cannot fit in and may have to go.

3 Where there are not enough resources such as money (inequality in pay between staff groups, for instance, leads to rivalry and hostility), time (e.g. lack of senior management time to support and encourage), space (not having enough room to do a variety of things, etc.) and status and position (e.g. not everyone can be in charge). These are often more difficult to resolve but creative and imaginative thinking may reduce some stresses by, for example, different organization of rotas or changing the use of some rooms.

4 When people exercise power and authority it can cause resentment. One way to reduce problems is to ensure that there are clear job descriptions. Everyone should know what they are responsible for and to whom they are responsible for doing it. If the lines of command are clear there should be fewer points of conflict. Chemistry does, however, play its part: people sometimes do find it difficult to exercise or respond to authority and managers need to be alert to potential difficulties.

5 The way things are organized may cause conflict. The allocation of tasks, for instance, may be seen as unfair. Meetings can be used to explain why some arrangements are necessary and for discussing other ways of doing things.

From a more positive point of view, all staff are employed because they have skills and abilities. The successful team will be the one that is able to use its members' skills most effectively. If people are given clear guidance and a system of beliefs with which they are in sympathy to guide them, they can then be given the autonomy to get on with their job in the most effective way they can. Delegation in this way enables people to develop their own strengths and is more likely to lead to creativity and new ideas.

Arranging the work

One of the most demanding tasks for managers in residential Homes is arranging time. This needs to be done in two senses. First, managers must arrange rotas to ensure that staff are available at the most necessary times; second, they must also arrange their own personal work time to the best advantage.

Rotas can be used to staff advantage. Recruitment is very difficult in some areas, much easier in others. Part-timers offer advantages of flexibility. It is easier to arrange a rota to ensure higher numbers of staff when the demands are greatest (early mornings, mealtimes, etc.) if there is a larger pool of part-time staff. On the other hand, larger numbers of people who only work a few hours a week make it more difficult to create a cohesive team, to arrange meetings, to provide training and therefore generally to provide a consistent approach to helping residents. A balance has to be struck between competing possibilities. It is essential to review rotas regularly to check whether they work to the residents' best advantage. It is easy for patterns and habits of work to develop around staff needs and wishes and a periodic, objective review of whether these also meet residents' needs is necessary.

Earlier there was some discussion of group living and how smaller groups of residents may be used within the wider life of the Home. These arrangements may be used to allocate to a small group of staff a particular commitment to those residents and their individual needs.

Another widely discussed and implemented approach has been called the 'key-worker approach'. The idea of a key worker – someone who takes the main responsibility for co-ordinating work and generally making sure that a client gets all she needs and is entitled to – developed first in field social work. In residential

Homes it has generally meant the same thing but it has actually been put into practice in very different ways.

Sometimes one care assistant is responsible for work with three or four residents, looking after their clothes, helping to bathe them, helping them with shopping, writing letters, etc. This approach has often been found unsatisfactory because the key worker is available only for a minority of the week. Others have tried attaching two key workers to a group of residents, or establishing larger teams of care workers with responsibilities to a group of residents.

There is little evidence that any one type of key-worker system is, alone, effective in providing a more individual approach. What is most important in both key-worker and group-living arrangements is that staff recognize and respond to individual needs and are concerned with resident need first and the convenience of themselves and the 'systems' of the Home second. Some Homes have found key-worker and/or group-living approaches work *for them* as effective ways of arranging their work to achieve this individualized approach. The essential thing is that staff teams take time to decide what will be the best ways for them and the residents with whom they work.

Whatever the system adopted, staff need to pass day-to-day information to each other about the business of the Home or about individual residents. This is usually done in two main ways: by written report books or sheets or cards for each resident, and by verbal hand-over sessions between shifts. Effective hand-over requires a commitment of time. If one shift ends at 2 p.m. and the next starts at 2 p.m. then there can be no effective discussion between different staff groups. There should be an overlap during which information can be given to incoming staff about the needs of residents and current events, as necessary, during face-to-face discussion. This should be backed up by written records.

Getting the best out of staff

The first stage in creating a good team of workers is selection. Recruiting the right people is essential. In order to do this it will be necessary to decide on the job to be done. There should be a clear job description which sets out the main aims of the job, the tasks that will be required, whom the worker will be accountable to and conditions of service – the rewards and limitations.

The next step will be deciding what sort of person: what attributes, skills and experience would be ideal for the job. This will then point to ways of advertising and places to put adverts to attract the right applicants. Interviewing is a skilled task in itself: decide who should be involved in the interview and whether to involve the applicants in visiting the Home and meeting the residents and other staff. Different styles will be right for different jobs. A half-hour interview by two or three people is not the best way to choose a senior Home manager. People show their true abilities (and inabilities) in different kinds of situations, and a variety of contacts during the selection process may be worth considering. Since it is the residents who will be most affected by a new Head of Home, for instance, they should have a chance to comment on what sort of person they want and to meet applicants.

Once appointed, new staff need a proper introduction to the Home and the job. In the first few days practicalities may be most important: finding their way around, learning what to do if there is a fire, accident procedures, lunch, tea or coffee breaks and what the job involves. For most staff the simple experience of 'being next to Nellie' will be enough in the first few days. This should, however, be linked to a basic induction experience. At the very least this should include, for care staff, an introduction to basic skills, monitored and supported by a manager. Preferably, it should include a series of on- and off-the-job experiences. An induction programme could include such things as receiving new residents, first aid, confidentiality, personal care tasks (e.g. dressing, bathing, toileting), hygiene, use of self-help equipment, introduction to mental disorder, death and dying. In particular, every opportunity should be taken to discuss the 'why' of working with people as well as the 'what' and 'how'. The reasons why particular approaches are important – the basic values and attitudes – come first.

Staff of all levels should have a routine opportunity to consider, with a senior manager, whether they have the skills to do their job properly and whether they wish to develop skills to fit them for promotion. Training and development are essential and should be based on a plan for each individual member of staff.

A major area of work for managers and staff is supervising and being supervised. Dealing with infirm, confused, sometimes aggressive and hostile and frequently very dependent elderly people is very demanding. In order to be able to separate themselves from the needs of residents and to make more objective assessments, workers need to be able to examine themselves and their reactions in discussions with colleagues – not necessarily administrative superiors.

Most discussions of 'supervision' in social work have been developed in relation to field social work where it includes matters to do with organizing work but also involves an opportunity to reflect on the progress of work – often emotionally demanding – with a colleague. The residential setting is very different from field social work. Everyone shares the same working situation and much of what is happening is visible to everyone in what has been called 'the life-space situation'. Supervision may often take the form of on-the-spot reaction, discussion or control. Support can be given, for instance, during or immediately after an emotional or hostile exchange or a mistake can be corrected at the time. In addition, time should be set aside for each worker to discuss with a manager his or her progress, current work and objectives and to consider better ways of doing the job.

Social services agencies have begun to recognize that social work in any setting is potentially stressful. Residential work with elderly people has its own pressures: people die, residents can be aggressive and even violent, and other staff can create stress. Different people are threatened, or 'stressed' by different things and at different times: events at home in the family or changes in health, for instance, can reduce thresholds of coping. Managers need to be alert to things that create stress (including, and perhaps especially, those in themselves). Some important considerations will be:

- to watch for what individuals find difficult to deal with;
- to be clear about the expectations of staff;
- to be clear about who is responsible;
- sometimes it will be right to seek help from outside the Home, from colleagues, managers or independent counsellors: stress is a part of everyone's work and good management involves helping to deal with it in a variety of ways.

Recording

Written records are essential in the Home for many reasons. They store information. They communicate information. They structure information.

Records are a necessary part of running the business. They indicate whether activities are meeting planned targets by, for example, giving finanacial information about whether there is overspending on budgets. They provide a reference if something goes wrong. Routine records of what happens each day in the Home are usually kept in logbooks. These may refer to individual residents and to events of the day. They should not include subjective comment ('Mr Jones was grumpy today') or disrespectful comment ('Mr Jones was a nuisance today'). It should be possible to transfer notes about each resident to individual files, which should be orderly and systematic. A good personal record should be accurate, up-to-date and relevant: it has always been good practice to share what is on a file with a resident unless there is a very good reason not to do so. The law now requires this if residents request it.

Records should be confidential. A daily logbook should be kept in a secure place, not left casually in an accessible area. Files should only be available to those staff who have a good reason to see the information in them.

Above all, good individual records maintain a commitment to the continuing progress of a resident's life. They should provide a basis for regular review and should include a note of key events, including such things as dental, hearing and eyesight tests (which should be regularly available). Life in a Home should not be static: it should include opportunities for change, activity and development. These should have a planned rationale which will be helped and clarified by routine recording. It is sometimes argued that when staff time is scarce, then written records are a luxury. This is not so: records are an *essential* tool of organized, coherent and consistent residential work practice.

GETTING IT RIGHT: QUALITY, STANDARDS AND ACCOUNTABILITY

A concern for the quality of the end product and ways of creating management systems and structures to achieve quality has been an increasingly prominent feature in both commercial and public sectors. Quality basically refers to whether or not a service (or product) actually achieves the purposes for which it is intended. In the present context that means whether or not the Home is doing what it should.

How will we judge Homes?

In order to decide whether a Home is doing well or not we need to have some standards or criteria by which to judge it. The authority on which standards are based comes from a number of sources: from statutory sources (the law and regulations); from ethical and moral values; from organizational (including governmental) rules (an important distinction will be between rules and guidelines, both of which may play a part in judging and measuring standards of performance); and from professional sources expressed in various ways, through common practice, professional associations, academic texts, etc.

There will, therefore, be different sorts of standards. They will include the most general rules which might be called 'ethical standards': this refers to basic principles of practice or values. There will also be technical or design standards which specify the explicit details of how a system or process or design is to be set up and carried out. These may also be called 'operational rules' or 'design guidance'. A further sort of standard might be called 'performance standards': these relate actions and resources to actual outcomes and are therefore more likely to stimulate creativity in the search for more effective or efficient ways of achieving the same outcome.

We do have some standards for Homes for elderly people available to us. Some categories of standards do, of course, lend themselves more readily to setting a range in which services can be judged to be adequate, good, excellent, etc. For example, ethical standards may be 'sound' or 'not sound' (it is difficult, for instance, to be 'fairly confidential'). Technical standards, however, may offer more scope for setting an acceptable range (e.g. 'Rooms should be at least 10.5 square metres but more comfort would be provided in rooms 50 per cent larger than this'). When we are thinking about standards, therefore, we need to be clear about whether we are looking for things to be good or 'good enough'.

The standards already available to us are not all easy to get at. There is some central government guidance but this tends to be advisory or outdated. *Local Authority Building Note 2*, for example, provides guidelines for design of Homes. It was issued in 1973 and, in 1986, *DHSS Circular LAC (86)1* confirmed that it would not be revised and recommended 'a flexible approach to design and operational policies'. Similarly, *Residential Homes for the Elderly. Arrangements for Health Care. A Memorandum of Guidance* (DHSS/ Welsh Office 1977), referred to earlier, is to be subject to review so that it now forms general guidance rather than clear standards.

Home Life (Centre for Policy on Ageing 1984) forms, together with the regulations associated with the Registered Homes Act (1984), the most specific set of standards currently available. It sets out broad principles of care – fulfilment, dignity, autonomy, individuality, esteem, quality of experience, emotional needs, risk and choice. These offer ethical standards: a general statement of values from which more detailed prescriptions can flow.

Local Authorities have developed their own packages of guidance for registration and inspection of Homes in the independent sector. These are generally derived from *Home Life*, DHSS guidance and various other sources (health and safety, fire legislation, etc.). Authorities vary widely in the extent to which they have adopted *Home Life* or any other standards in any explicit form for their own Homes.

It is also possible to look to training, professional and research sources for indications of generally accepted or understood standards. Many of these have been introduced earlier in the book.

Whatever standards we use should themselves be able to stand up to challenge. They will need to be justifiable, as precise and therefore measurable as possible, practical and real (they must work in practice and relate to real life). They must also be realistic in recognizing the lack of resources and they must be acceptable in the political, organizational and professional situations in which they will be used.

Who will judge standards? Inspection, management and accountability

The system for regulating Homes in the independent sector was laid down by the Registered Homes Act (1984). Homes with four or more people requiring board and personal care must be registered (with some special exceptions) with the Local Authority. Once registered, they receive a certificate which specifies the numbers of people they can provide for and may make special conditions about their age and sex.

In Local Authorities' own Homes, arrangements for monitoring the quality of the service to residents vary. In many this is seen as the responsibility of the line-manager, who may carry out a formal inspection or review on a regular basis or may rely on routine, informal visits. A number of Social Services Departments have developed inspection teams which are separate from the line of management and which carry out regular, formal inspection visits or spot-checks on particular Homes. The 1989 White Paper Proposes the setting up of such 'arm's-length' inspection units in all Social Services Departments.

To date experience seems to have been of broadly three types of approach, although with very blurred dividing lines:

1 Management reviews, carried out by line-managers to inform themselves in greater detail about current issues, to review goals set previously and to set new targets. Often these are carried out as joint development exercises with the staff (and sometimes residents) of the Homes.
2 Inspections within the organization's own structure but done as a check on standards by one or more workers separate from line-management.
3 Inspections by people from outside the agency: usually Local Authority inspectors but occasionally by consultants called in by Local Authority Homes or by the Social Services Inspectorate of the Department of Health.

Inspectors get information from two main sources. First, from discussions and observations on visits to Homes and from papers provided before and during visits. Second, from informal and indirect channels: complaints, social workers, obituary columns, newspaper ads, etc. The quality of an inspection depends on the reliability, detail and accuracy of the information available. It also depends on the way in which the information is put together to give it meaning and relate it to agreed standards.

In the midst of these developing systems of inspection and monitoring, the manager of the Home has a key position. Inspection and review visits can fulfil at least three purposes:

1 They provide a routine check on whether the Home meets the basic requirements and criteria. They are a regulating mechanism.
2 They are an opportunity to influence practice in the Home. They have a developmental function.
3 They are a means of confirming that there is no unacceptable practice in the Home. They are a way of picking up on abuses.

The Head of Home, like other staff, will need support and super-vision. This is usually provided in the Local Authority by the line-manager, although management control of aspects of building, personnel and finance may well involve other sections of the department or even other departments of the Local Authority. In smaller private Homes both professional care supervision and business management control or support are less likely to be available and Associations of Proprietors have been formed, in part to offer mutual support and assistance across the range of tasks to be done.

The Head of Home is responsible for 'getting it right' but is accountable to others for the rightness of practice. That account-ability is, in one sense, to line-managers but in another sense it is to the person or agency that is regulating standards. At least as important is the accountability to the residents: they are the customers, the purchasers of service.

Inspection and quality checking (including the checks made by buildings, fire, health, hygiene and safety personnel) have become central elements of residential care for elderly people. A con-sciousness of quality (of the importance of making sure the service does what it is supposed to do and meets consumers' needs) should pervade all management action. The demands and skills of inspecting and being inspected need to be a part of residential work thinking in all its dimensions, whether management or professional care practice.

GETTING IT WRONG: WHISTLE-BLOWING AND COMPLAINTS

Bad things do happen in institutions. These can range from the thoughtless to the vicious and cruel. There has been a long series of inquiries into allegations of bad practice and ill-treatment in institutions in the last 30 years. Some of the more significant have been Robb's *Sans Everything* (1967), which was an informal description of abuses in long-stay hospitals, and a number of formal inquiries into psychiatric and geriatric hospitals in the 1960s and early 1970s (e.g. Ely Report 1969; Farleigh Report 1971; Whittingham Report 1972), through to a number of independent inquiries into practices in residential Homes in London and elsewhere in the late 1980s.

Evidence to the Wagner Committee confirms that cruelty and neglect occur. In a review of the evidence to the committee, E. Sinclair (1988) notes that 16 out of 105 judgements made by residents and 23 out of 100 views from residents and others were totally negative. There were allegations of deliberate cruelty: a lady of 98 being tipped out of her wheelchair; residents being teased or frightened; a resident, who was doubly incontinent, and being humiliated by 'the care assistant, who 'gathered it up in white tissue and wiped it across the resident's face'(p.139). More common were allegations of extreme neglect, including serious delays in treatment and residents being locked in rooms or chairs. Sinclair (p.146) lists factors in Homes about which the correspondents appeared to be unhappy. These are important and worth repeating in full:

Cruelty, ill-treatment or neglect are over-looked by those in charge.

Admission has not resulted from a resident's own considered decision.

Regimes are designed for the convenience of an inadequate staff rather than to maintain the comfort of residents.

Activities and outings are few or non-existent.

Visitors are not made welcome.

Food, furnishings and facilities are poor.

There is no respect for residents' dignity, individual personality or ability.

Conversation, shared enjoyment and affection are not valued or enjoyed.

It is very difficult for individual members of staff to affect situations of substantial or long-standing abuse of this nature. 'Whistle-blowing', or making serious complaints about bad practice, is very difficult. There are strong pressures within Homes to conform to usual patterns of behaviour. These may not include overt and explicit abuse but may lead to consistent deprivation and disrespect for residents over a long period. A junior member of staff may be powerless to create any change and will usually feel vulnerable in making a complaint, may not know who to complain to anyway, and may feel uncertain about whether or not some things would be regarded as wrong by senior managers or independent inspectors.

Similarly, it may be difficult for relatives to complain because of fear that it may lead to worse repercussions for the resident and perhaps because of anxiety that the alternative may be to take on the care of the elderly person themselves. Residents are in the most vulnerable position of all: they depend on staff help, sometimes even to the extent of enabling them to articulate or write, so they are unable to complain without some staff co-operation.

The Head of Home is usually the most powerful person in such situations. Sometimes, however, a long-established staff group can obstruct attempts by new managers to create necessary change. It should not be assumed that the Head of Home is always the one controlling bad practice. It may be that she is colluding and enables it to continue through inability to find a way of changing things.

One way to reduce the chance of abuse is to create a formal complaints system (as opposed to a staff grievance procedure). This should tell staff, residents, relatives and others about how a complaint should be made if there are problems about care in the Home. This information needs to be readily available and should be included in initial information to new staff and residents. The Registered Homes Act (1984) requires that residents be told how and where to make a complaint and it is good practice for Local Authorities to do the same.

There should also be an agreed way of dealing with complaints. Many will go informally to the Head of Home in the first place and can be dealt with amicably through discussion. A written record should be kept of all but the most minor ones and senior managers or inspectors should see the records routinely. More serious complaints may be dealt with by senior managers or Local Authority inspectors. Allegations should be investigated carefully, written statements taken wherever possible and a written report made to the responsible authority with recommendations for action. It is sensible, in the most serious cases, for someone outside the line of management to investigate.

Any complaints system is only as good as the system for putting things right where there are found to be faults. When things have gone wrong, a senior management decision will need to be made about what action needs to be taken and who should take it. This should be made clear to all concerned, including – and especially – the person making the complaint. There should be a built-in check at a specified time to confirm that action has been taken and changes made.

Complaint systems will only work, however, if people feel confident that something positive will happen if they do complain. Fear of reprisals can be strong (and realistically so). Managers and Homes inspectors should make themselves known to residents and should be regularly 'visible' in the Homes. If they can build up an atmosphere of trust, and encourage staff, residents and their relatives to believe that they are available to help and respond, there may be a greater willingness to complain if necessary.

The best way of dealing with complaints, of course, is to make sure there is nothing to complain about! Since you can never please all of the people all of the time in any group, expect some dissatisfaction; try not to respond defensively and certainly not aggressively; and listen and try to understand what people want.

CONSUMER SATISFACTION AND ADVOCACY

Staff may not always be the best people to help residents with some problems. The influence of institutional systems is strong and it is sometimes difficult to find the time and objectivity to respond to individuals within the pressures of daily work and group demands.

It is difficult to get an accurate picture of what residents truly feel and want. They typically express satisfaction with the present situation, perhaps because they are reluctant to complain, perhaps because they cannot imagine alternatives, but perhaps because they are genuinely satisfied. Not all residents want the same things, of course, so attempts to consult with the resident group as a whole may produce different results from consultations with individuals. It is, however, important that residents be enabled to express their views freely and seek satisfaction for their needs: quite simply because they have a right to do so.

Managers should use a variety of ways of seeking residents' views – by group discussion, formal and informal contacts with individual residents; and, from time to time, it may be useful to carry out structured research across a resident population to consider their wishes and feelings in more depth. Some experiments have involved more able elderly people living for a short time in a Home, specifically to report to managers on the experience.

One potential approach is to use advocates to work with individual residents to make sure they get all they have a right to and a fair share of the resources available. Much of the development of thinking about advocacy in the UK has been based on work with people with mental handicaps living in hospitals. Advocacy has been defined in the following terms (Sang and O'Brien 1984: 9):

> Advocacy occurs when a private citizen enters into a relationship with, and represents the interests of a mentally handicapped person who needs assistance to improve his or her quality of life and obtain full rights and entitlements. By providing emotional support through friendship, spokespersonship, opportunities to learn new skills, and help in obtaining needed services, volunteers work for the benefit and growth of people who are handicapped.

This definition refers primarily to when a lay person enters into a relationship with someone in an institution in order to assist them. There seems to be no reason why the definition should not apply to elderly residents. There are, of course, all sorts of advocacy: helping residents to assert their own rights; legal advocacy; financial advocacy; and formal guardianship arrangements which may involve a legal element.

One particularly difficult area is the management of financial affairs where the residents appear to be confused. *Home Life* (Centre for Policy on Ageing 1984: 65) recommends:

> In the absence of someone known to the resident the registration authority should be asked to recommend someone to act as agent. References for agents should be sought, and all names of individuals and organizations acting as agents should be lodged with the registration authority. Only in

exceptional circumstances should the proprietor or manager assume the role of agent.

There is actually little evidence of any widespread use of agents or advocates in Homes for elderly people. This is an important area for development and one which staff should be enabled to see as positive and enhancing residents' rights rather than as threatening or undermining to their own position and control. Advocacy seems to have been most successful where groups of volunteer advocates have been given training and support.

BRINGING IT ALL TOGETHER: KEY POINTS

The most important person in a Home is generally its manager: the Head of Home or Officer-in-Charge. She is responsible for making sure all the diverse tasks and needs come together to make a good Home. These tasks fall into three main areas of creating and maintaining a suitable building; running the business; and providing personal and social care in a homely environment.

The important issues for managing these tasks are the need to provide a clear statement of values and to enable staff to accept and understand the implications of these; to provide clear guidelines on what good care involves but to give staff sufficient autonomy to develop and use their own skills and strengths; and to find a balance between valuing staff and residents and working constructively with areas of tension between the needs of each group.

A commitment to quality is essential: both quality of care, practices and resources, and quality of life as measured by consumer satisfaction. Standards should be explicit so people know how they will be judged. Inspection can be a regulating mechanism to ensure things are 'good enough' but also can and should be used positively to improve and develop.

Sometimes things go wrong. There should ideally be good information about how and where to make complaints and, especially, management systems for 'righting wrongs' and checking that things have been put right.

One way to check whether problems are occurring is to provide a variety of ways of listening to elderly residents who are often reluctant to say that they are not satisfied. One important area for development is the use of advocates, with appropriate training and support.

WHERE TO LEARN MORE

There is little written about management in residential Homes for elderly people. Two works may be helpful in some areas of practice:

Whitton, J.R. (1982) *Managing to Care*, Hayle, Cornwall: The Patten Press.

Hooper, B. (1984) *Home Ground. How to Select and Get the Best Out of Staff*, Centre for Policy on Ageing.

The second of these is a loose-leaf handbook about staff support and training. *In Search of Excellence* (Peters and Waterman 1982) is a lively and enthusiastic approach to managing for quality.
On selecting and developing staff:

Kahan, B., Banner, G. and Lane, D. (1986) *Staff. . . Finding Them. . . Choosing Them. . . Keeping Them*, Surbiton, Surrey: SCA Publications.

On standards and inspection:

Kellaher, L. *et al.* (1988) *Coming to Terms with the Private Sector. Report No. I: Public Sector Responses to the Private Sector*, London: PNL Press.

On whistle-blowing:

Beardshaw, V. (1981) *Conscientious Objectors at Work. Mental Hospital Nurses: A Case Study*, London: Social Audit Ltd.

On advocacy: Sang and O'Brien (1984), referred to in the text, give a general review of issues.

Chapter Nine

REFLECTIONS: A FINAL WORD

There is no easy way of providing a concise summary of all that this book has covered. There is a note of the key points at the end of each chapter which should highlight the most important things. If anything needs special stress it is:

1 *Be purposeful:* be clear about why you are doing something and who you are doing it for. Make sure everyone else understands it too: communicate, share information.
2 *Get the attitudes right:* be clear about the values that underlie and justify what you are doing.
3 *See people as individuals:* listen to what they say and assess what they need. People cannot always have what they want but do make sure they get their fair share.

Residential provision in the late 1980s has been in a state of change. In 1989 a Government White Paper (Dept of Health 1989) set out a wide range of plans for the organization of community care services. Among other things, it heralded changes in the way in which financial support would be given to elderly people for residential care. It proposed new arrangements for assessment for and management of care services, and it set out new arrangements for quality control of Local Authority Homes. Potentially it set an agenda for radical changes in the organization, purchasing, provision and monitoring of residential care.

The future offers many prospects and potentials for different kinds of permanent and non-permanent accommodation with support and care help for elderly people. Issues for the future include:

- Where will residential care be provided: public- or independent-sector balance? How will systems of quality checking develop as they begin to apply equally across both sectors?
- How will the shifts in arrangements to pay for residential care affect the balance of provision and the rights of elderly people?
- How will multi-disciplinary assessment develop to offer assessment to all people who go into Homes and how to ensure they all know the options?
- What sort of Homes will there be: big or small? Group-living arrangements? Specialist? Other?
- How will resource centres develop: providing a variety of support, including accommodation for elderly people in a locality?
- How can short-term residential and other kinds of respite care be developed? Rotating care? Specialist units? Other?
- How will changes in community care provisions affect the use of Homes? What sort of people will need residential Homes in the future?
- How can appropriate staff be recruited, trained and supported?

There are exciting and important issues and changes: it would take another book to consider them properly. For many of these questions, only time will tell.

BIBLIOGRAPHY

ADSS (1986) *Evidence of the Association of Directors of Social Services: Review of Residential Care*, London: ADSS.

Age Concern England (1989) *Guidelines for Setting Up Advocacy Schemes*, London: Age Concern England.

Allen, I. (1983) *Short-stay Residential Care for the Elderly*, London: Policy Studies Institute.

Audit Commission (1985) *Managing Social Services for the Elderly More Effectively*, London: HMSO.

Barton, R. (1959) *Institutional Neurosis*, Bristol: John Wright.

Berry, J. (1972) 'The experience of reception into residential care', *British Journal of Social Work*, 2(4): 423–34.

Birren, J.E. (1986) 'The process of aging', in A. Pifer and L. Bronte (eds) *Our Aging Society: Paradox and Promise*, New York: Norton.

Booth, T. (1985) *Home Truths: Old People's Homes and the Outcomes of Care*, Aldershot: Gower.

Booth, T. and Phillips, D. (1987) 'Group living in homes for the elderly: a comparative study of the outcomes of care', *British Journal of Social Work* 17: 1–20.

Briggs, A. and Oliver, J. (1985) *Caring: Experiences of Looking After Disabled Relatives*, London: Routledge & Kegan Paul.

Buckingham, G., Dimmock, B. and Truscott, D. (1979) *Beyond Tea, Bingo and Condescension*, Stoke-on-Trent: Beth Johnson Foundation/Task Force.

Centre for Policy on Ageing (1984) *Home Life: A Code of Practice for Residential Care*, London.

Cooper, J. (1980) *Social Groupwork with Elderly People in Hospital*, Stoke-on-Trent: Beth Johnson Foundation.

Davies, B. and Knapp, M. (1981) *Old People's Homes and the Production of Welfare*, London: Routledge & Kegan Paul.

Department of Health (1989) *Caring for People. Community Care in the Next Decade and Beyond*, cmnd 849, London: HMSO.

DHSS/Welsh Office (1973) *Local Authority Building Note 2. Residential Accommodation for Elderly People,* London: HMSO.

DHSS/Welsh Office (1977) *Residential Homes for the Elderly. Arrangements for Health Care. A Memorandum of Guidance,* London: HMSO.

DHSS (1981) *Growing Older,* cmnd 8173, London: HMSO.

DHSS (1986) *Residential Homes—Guidance on Standards of Accommodation,* Circular LAC(86)1.

Ely Report (1969) *Report of the Committee of Inquiry into Allegations of Ill-treatment of Patients at Ely Hospital,* cmnd 3975, London: HMSO.

Erikson, E. (1964) *Childhood and Society,* rev. edn, New York: Norton.

Evans, D. *et al.* (1981) *The Management of Mental and Physical Impairment in Non-specialist Residential Homes for the Elderly,* University of Manchester.

Farleigh Report (1971) *Report of the Farleigh Hospital Committee of Inquiry,* cmnd 4557, London: HMSO.

Ford, J. and Sinclair, R. (1987) *Sixty Years On. Women Talk about Old Age,* London: The Women's Press.

Fry, M. (1954) *Old Age Looks at Itself,* London: National Old People's Welfare Council.

Gearing, B., Johnson, M. and Heller, T. (eds) (1988) *Mental Health Problems in Old Age,* New York: John Wiley & Sons

Gibberd, K. (1977) *Home for Life. Residential Care. What Alternatives?,* London: Age Concern England.

Gibbs, I. and Bradshaw, J. (1987a) 'How much?' *Social Services Insight,* 7 August 1987: 18–20.

Gibbs, I. and Bradshaw, J. (1987b) 'Who needs assessment?' *Community Care,* December 1987: 24.

Goffman, E. (1961) *Asylums. Essays on the Social Situation of Mental Patients and Other Inmates,* New York: Doubleday.

Goldberg, E. M. and Connelly, N. (1982) *The Effectiveness of Social Care for the Elderly,* London: Heinemann.

Goodrich, E. K. (1976) 'My experience of deafness', *Deafness and the Elderly,* London: Age Concern Greater London.

Gray, B. and Isaacs, B. (1979) *Care of the Elderly Mentally Infirm,* London: Tavistock Publications.

Green, H. (1988) *Informal Carers. General Household Survey, 1985,* London: HMSO.

Griffiths, R. (1988) *Community Care: Agenda for Action,* London: HMSO.

Harris, A. I. (1968) *Social Welfare for the Aged,* London: HMSO.

Hunt, A. (1978) *The Elderly at Home,* London: HMSO.

Ingersoll, B. and Silverman, A. (1978) 'Comparative group psychotherapy for the aged', *Gerontologist* 18(2): 201–6.

Jones, K. (1972) 'The twenty-four steps: an analysis of institutional admission procedures', *Sociology* 6: 405–14.

Jones, K. and Fowles, A. J. (1984) *Ideas on Institutions: Analysing the Literature on Long-term Care and Custody*, London: Routledge & Kegan Paul.

Joseph, J. (1974) 'Warning', from *Rose in the Afternoon*, London: Dent.

Judge, K. and Sinclair, I. (eds) (1986) *Residential Care for Elderly People* London: HMSO.

Judge, K. *et al.* (1986) 'The comparative costs of public and private residential homes for the elderly', in K. Judge and I. Sinclair (eds) *Residential Care for Elderly People*, London: HMSO.

Lawrence, S. *et al.* (1987) *She's Leaving Home*, Polytechnic of North London.

Lawton, M. P. (1980) *Environment and Aging*, California: Wadsworth Inc.

Lipman, A. and Slater, R. (1977) 'Homes for old people: towards a positive environment', *Gerontologist* 17: 146–56.

McCall, R. (1979) *Communication Barriers in the Elderly*, London: Age Concern England.

McCormack, P. (date unknown) 'Look closer', quoted in B. Kerr (1985) *She'd Be Better Off in a Home...Wouldn't She?*, London: Central Council for Education and Training in Social Work (CCETSW) Paper 3.1.

Mandelstam, D. (1985) 'Incontinence', in M. Hawker *The Older Patient and the Role of the Physiotherapist*, London: Faber & Faber.

Martin, D. and Peckford, B. (1978) 'Hearing impairment in homes for the elderly', *Social Work Service* 17: 52–62.

Martin, J., Meltzer, H. and Elliot, D. (1988) *The Prevalence of Disability among Adults*, London: HMSO.

Ministry of Health (1955) *Circular 3/55*, London: HMSO.

Ministry of Health (1957) *Circular 14/57*, London: HMSO.

Ministry of Health (1965) *Circular 18/65*, London: HMSO.

National Institute for Social Work (1988) *Residential Care for Elderly People: Using Research to Improve Practice*, London: NISW.

Norman, A. (1984) *Bricks and Mortals*, London: Centre for Policy on Ageing.

Norman, A. (1987a) *Severe Dementia: The Provision of Long-stay Care*, London Centre for Policy on Ageing.

Norman, A. (1987b) *Aspects of Ageism: A Discussion Paper*, London: Centre for Policy on Ageing.

Parker, R. (1988) 'Residential care', in I. Sinclair (1988) *Residential Care Reviewed*, London: NISW/HMSO.

Peace, S. *et al.* (1982) *A Balanced Life?*, Polytechnic of North London.

Peace, S. (1986) 'The design of residential homes: an historical perspective', in K. Judge and I. Sinclair (eds) *Residential Care for Elderly People*, London: HMSO.

Peters, T. J. and Austin, N. (1985) *A Passion for Excellence: The Leadership Difference*, London: Collins.

Peters, T. J. and Waterman, R. H. (1982) *In Search of Excellence*, New York: Harper & Row.

Phillips Committee (1954) *Report of the Committee on the Economic and Financial Problems of the Provision for Old Age*, cmnd 9333, London: HMSO.

Pope, P. (1978) 'Admissions to residential homes for the elderly', *Social Work Today* 9(44): 12–16.

Rees, S. (1978) *Social Work Face to Face*, London: Edward Arnold.

Robb, B. (1967) *Sans Everything: A Case to Answer*, Walton-on-Thames: Nelson.

Sang, B. and O'Brien, J. (1984) *Advocacy: The UK and American Experience*, London: Kings Fund Centre, project paper 51.

Schmidt, P. (1931) *The Conquest of Old Age*, London: George Routledge & Sons.

Scrutton, S. (1989) *Counselling Older People*, London: Edward Arnold.

Seabrook, J. (1980) *The Way We Are: Old People Talk about Themselves*, London: Age Concern England.

Seligman, M.E.P. and Maier S. F. (1967) 'Failure to escape traumatic shock', *Journal of Experimental Psychology* 74: 1–9.

Sinclair, E. (1988) *Guide to the Evidence. Appendix 1 to A Positive Choice (Wagner Report)*, London: NISW/HMSO.

Sinclair, I. (1986) 'The residents: characteristics and reasons for admission', in K. Judge and I. Sinclair (eds) *Residential Care for Elderly People*, London: HMSO.

Sinclair, I. (ed.) (1988) *Residential Care. The Research Reviewed*, London: NISW/HMSO.

Slack, P. and Mulville, F. (1987) *Sweet Adeline. A Journey Through Care*, Basingstoke: Macmillan Education.

Slater, R. and Lipman, A. (1976) 'Accommodation options for old people: towards an operational philosophy', *Design for Special Needs: Journal of the Centre on Environment for the Handicapped* 11: 10–15.

Social Services Inspectorate, DHSS (1988) *Say it Again. Contemporary Social Work Practice with People Who Are Deaf or Hard of Hearing*, London: DHSS.

Sontag, S. (1972) 'The double standard of aging', in V. Carver and P. Liddiard (eds) (1978) *An Ageing Population*, London: Hodder & Stoughton.

Standing Conference of Ethnic Minority Citizens (1988) *Making a Reality of Residential Care for Ethnic Minority Elderly*, London: Standing Conference of Ethnic Minority Citizens.

Stott, M. (1981) *Ageing for Beginners*, Oxford: Basil Blackwell.

Tobin, S. and Lieberman, M. A. (1976) *Last Home for the Aged*, California: Jossey-Bass.

Townsend, P. (1962) *The Last Refuge*, London: Routledge & Kegan Paul.

Wagner Report (1988) *Residential Care. A Positive Choice*, London: NISW/HMSO.

Weaver, T. *et al.* (1985) *The Business of Care: A Study of Private Residential Homes for Old People*, Polytechnic of North London.

Whittingham Report (1972) *Report of the Committee of Inquiry into Whittingham Hospital*, cmnd 4861, London: HMSO.

Willcocks, D. *et al.* (1982) *The Residential Life of Old People: A Study in 100 Local Authority Old People's Homes*, vol. 1 Research Report no.12, Survey Research Unit, Polytechnic of North London.

Willcocks, D. *et al.* (1987) *Private Lives in Public Places*, London: Tavistock Publications.

NAME INDEX

SUBJECT INDEX